Dear Reader,
I did not become a doctor to get rich or famous.
Had I wanted those things, I would have chosen
another career path. I became a pediatrician
because I want to see all children growing up
happy and healthy. I want to spare them suffering
from infections, and I want to spare you the mental
anguish while caring for your sick children.

   We are embattled on two fronts—the threat of
infections and the menace of autism. One thing
needs to be completely clear. Doctors should work
with parents to combat these daunting foes. Parents
and doctors need to work together, not against each
other. Being united on the same team is the only
way that we have any chance of succeeding in
defeating these common enemies together.

   This book will hopefully serve as a unifying
force and help heal old wounds while building a
bright future for our children. We are in this
together. We need to be in this together.

Dr. Leslie Young

WELCOME TO THE

EVERYTHING®

PARENT'S GUIDES

Everything® Parent's Guides are a part of the bestselling *Everything*® series and cover common parenting issues like childhood illnesses and tantrums, as well as medical conditions like asthma and juvenile diabetes. These family-friendly books are designed to be a one-stop guide for parents. If you want authoritative information on specific topics not fully covered in other books, *Everything*® Parent's Guides are your perfect solution.

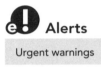 **Alerts**

Urgent warnings

 Facts

Important snippets of information

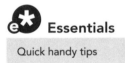 **Essentials**

Quick handy tips

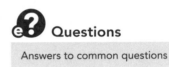 **Questions**

Answers to common questions

When you're done reading, you can finally say you know **EVERYTHING**®!

PUBLISHER Karen Cooper

DIRECTOR OF ACQUISITIONS AND INNOVATION Paula Munier

MANAGING EDITOR, EVERYTHING® SERIES Lisa Laing

COPY CHIEF Casey Ebert

ACQUISITIONS EDITOR Brett Palana-Shanahan

SENIOR DEVELOPMENT EDITOR Brett Palana-Shanahan

EDITORIAL ASSISTANT Hillary Thompson

EVERYTHING® SERIES COVER DESIGNER Erin Alexander

LAYOUT DESIGNERS Colleen Cunningham, Elisabeth Lariviere, Ashley Vierra, Denise Wallace

Visit the entire Everything® series at *www.everything.com*

THE

EVERYTHING®

PARENT'S GUIDE TO

VACCINES

Balanced, professional advice to help you
make the best decision for your child

Leslie Young, MD

Aadamsmedia

Avon, Massachusetts

I am dedicating this book to my wife, Sherry, and my son, Scott. My wife patiently supported me while I spent long weekends and nights writing this book, and my son motivates me to create a brighter future for all children.

An Everything® Series Book.
Everything® and everything.com® are registered trademarks of F+W Media, Inc.

Published by Adams Media, a division of F+W Media, Inc.
57 Littlefield Street, Avon, MA 02322 U.S.A.
www.adamsmedia.com

ISBN 10: 1-60550-366-5
ISBN 13: 978-1-60550-366-0

Printed in the United States of America.

10 9 8 7 6 5 4 3 2 1

Library of Congress Cataloging-in-Publication Data
is available from the publisher.

This publication is designed to provide accurate and authoritative information with regard to the subject matter covered. It is sold with the understanding that the publisher is not engaged in rendering legal, accounting, or other professional advice. If legal advice or other expert assistance is required, the services of a competent professional person should be sought.
—From a *Declaration of Principles* jointly adopted by a Committee of the American Bar Association and a Committee of Publishers and Associations

Many of the designations used by manufacturers and sellers to distinguish their products are claimed as trademarks. Where those designations appear in this book and Adams Media was aware of a trademark claim, the designations have been printed with initial capital letters.

The Everything© Parents Guide to Vaccines is intended as a reference volume only, not as a medical manual. In light of the complex, individual, and specific nature of health problems, this book is not intended to replace professional medical advice. The ideas, procedures, and suggestions in this book are intended to supplement, not replace, the advice of a trained medical professional. Consult your physician before adopting the suggestions in this book, as well as about any condition that may require diagnosis or medical attention. The author and publisher disclaim any liability arising directly or indirectly from the use of this book.

This book is available at quantity discounts for bulk purchases. For information, please call 1-800-289-0963.

All the examples and dialogues used in this book are fictional, and have been created by the author to illustrate particular situations.

Acknowledgments

I would like to thank the most important person in my life, my wife, Sherry. She has accommodated my busy work and writing schedule so I could complete this book on time. I also want to thank my son, Scott. He inspires me to be a better pediatrician, and he sat on my lap to motivate me as I wrote. I am grateful for the expertise offered by my dear friend Dr. Chuen-Yen Lau. She provided me with invaluable information from her experience working with the HIV vaccine. I appreciate the professional and personal input from the Sermo community. I also want to express gratitude to my agent, Gina, for offering me the opportunity to write this book and suggesting wonderful ideas along the way. Finally, I want to thank my editor, Brett, who assisted me in getting my ideas across in the most effective manner.

Contents

Introduction

Primum non nocere is a Latin phrase meaning "First do no harm." This is one of the first doctrines taught to new physicians in medical school. It is a sacred oath, and it reminds doctors to first consider any possible harm that might occur from any medical procedure before conducting any intervention for an illness. If a doctor fails to adhere to this dictum, it is negligence.

It is a fact that vaccines can trigger serious and sometimes life-threatening reactions. It is also true that vaccines have helped to eradicate many dangerous infections that used to be common. Faced with these incontrovertible facts, physicians are confronted with the daunting decision whether to immunize their patients. Parents must also decide whether immunization is the right thing to do for their children.

Immunization has become a controversial topic for many reasons. Parents are more savvy and information is more easily accessible with modern technology. In addition, consumers are more inclined to take control of their health care than to blindly follow the advice of health-care professionals. However, the vast quantity of readily available information has not simplified the decision-making process. Sometimes the information is outdated, and sometimes the information is inaccurate. It is often impossible to ascertain the reliability of the source of the information, especially if the information was obtained from the Internet. To determine which vaccine is safe and beneficial, it requires years of professional training and a scientific background.

This book is written to present reliable and up-to-date information on immunization from an unbiased perspective. Facts are presented to the readers in an easy-to-read format and without any technical jargon. Unlike many provaccine and antivaccine titles, there is no agenda for writing this book. Facts are presented without a bias, and the reader must weigh the information and make a personal choice on whether to get vaccinated.

Communities for and against immunization are passionate about what they believe. Devastating conditions, such as autism, have been attributed to vaccines. Consequently, the debates can create high tension between physicians and patients. Many doctors refuse to provide service to patients unless they agree to be vaccinated according to the standard immunization schedule. As a result, patients are forced to abandon their doctors and search for ones who will accommodate their needs. This is unfortunate, because at the end, doctors and patients are really after the same thing. Preserving good health is the goal of all physicians. There is nothing for doctors to gain if patients suffer from complications resulting from vaccines. The fact that there is a common goal between doctors and patients is often overlooked in the immunization controversy. This book will help you to look beyond the hype and emotions and study the matter with a clear head.

CHAPTER 1

A Historical Perspective

When vaccination was first invented, it was a crude and barbaric procedure. People were intentionally infected with germs, and if they did not die from the infection, they became protected from the infection for the rest of their life. The risks were high, and it was a highly controversial practice. Subsequent vaccination programs were wrought with problems and tragedy. Here is a look at how the modern vaccination program evolved over the years.

Before Immunization

Ever since the invention of the first vaccine, people have been suspicious of them. Contrary to traditional medical treatment, a vaccine is a medical intervention that is administered to healthy individuals—before they get sick. The very notion of injecting something foreign into the body that could be potentially harmful rubs many people the wrong way, and it also seems to go against common sense. Why should you receive treatment before you get sick?

The recent movement of parents questioning medical authority and deciding against vaccination for their children is nothing new. Historically, people have hesitated to participate in and demonized the role of community-wide immunization programs for hundreds of years. What is different in today's world is that information can be disseminated quickly and efficiently. But that information may be good or bad. It is often impossible to distinguish between reliable information and misguided information. Much of the misinformation is often circulated by people with good intentions.

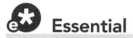 **Essential**

The goal of any vaccine is the total permanent elimination of a particular infection. It has already happened with smallpox, and it could happen with polio in the near future. It is likely that, with an effective global vaccination program, children of the future would need very few or no vaccines because diseases that we currently vaccinate against would no longer exist.

You can trace the history of vaccination in this country to the Colonial times and the Revolutionary War. In many ways, immunization and infection shaped this country into the way it is today.

Divine Intervention

Prior to the invention of vaccines, people approached illnesses differently. Getting sick was viewed mostly as a divine punishment for sins committed in the past. People sought medical as well as religious intervention for their illnesses. Also, poor sanitation and inadequate diets often meant children suffered the brunt of infectious disease outbreaks. Many children never had a chance to mature into adulthood, and parents accepted the death of their children because it was perceived as divine judgment (and there was little they could do to protect their children anyway).

Outbreaks of smallpox raged through towns and villages, claiming lives of friends and family. The fact that germs caused people to get sick wasn't discovered until more than 150 years after the first vaccination program. When an epidemic of infection struck a town, the only thing that could be done was to pray for the lives of loved ones. Each outbreak was an invisible enemy that seemed to randomly strike people. Thousands died with each infectious outbreak. Smallpox rivaled the Black Death in its impact on the population, and it was the leading cause of death in many cities.

 Fact

In the past, smallpox was a terrifying scourge that claimed millions of lives. Infections usually occurred in outbreaks, and smallpox would sweep through towns and villages, killing people of all ages. It was the number one cause of death for many parts of the world.

Of course, we now know that smallpox and other diseases are not the result of divine intervention. Germs are responsible for causing infections. You no longer have to pray to get well, and the availability of modern medicine offers many treatment options to beat back the invasion of germs. In addition, there are vaccines that help prevent the infection before you get sick. Many of the past scourges have become distant historical footnotes, including smallpox and polio. These infections seem as irrelevant in today's world as bleeding patients to cure a fever.

Return to the Past

Ironically, the historical past is fast becoming a reality in today's world. Due to concerns about vaccine safety, more and more parents today are electing to opt out of immunizing their children. A large number of school children no longer receive any vaccines at all because most schools allow parents to decline childhood immunization with a simple written statement. Just ask your friends and neighbors. Undoubtedly many of them will tell you that their children have never received any vaccine since birth.

The question now is whether smallpox and polio will make a comeback in a society where a large number of people are not vaccinated. Both of these infections are extremely rare now.

Smallpox is relegated to a few highly quarantined military laboratories. Smallpox's last victims died in 1978 as a result of an accidental laboratory exposure. Polio is limited to a handful of countries in the world—mainly India, a few countries in the Middle East, and some parts of Africa. Just over 1,000 cases of polio are being diagnosed a year. With so few circulating infections, can these germs still make a comeback if no one is immunized? At this point in time, no one knows the answer because it hasn't occurred. Most children are still immunized, even though that number is rapidly dwindling. What the future holds for these historical infections is anyone's guess. What is known is that, for the next few decades, the landscape for vaccination and infection will drastically change because more and more children are vaccine-free.

Alert

A phone survey conducted by the *Journal of the American Medical Association* in 2000 found that one in four American parents is reluctant to vaccinate their children. Consequently, a large number of children in school today have never received any immunization.

The Beginning

Vaccines have a humble beginning. Smallpox was the first infection that people tried to prevent. For more than a thousand years, the Chinese practiced an ancient form of vaccination by first grinding up the scabs from a person infected with smallpox, then blowing the powder into the nose of an unexposed individual. This practice is called *variolation,* and it originated from the observation that people who survived a previous smallpox infection somehow become resistant to getting the infection again. It was thought that by artificially infecting an unaffected person, the process could protect the individual from smallpox.

Ancient Chinese documents show that variolation was practiced in the Song dynasty in China (AD 960 to 1279). Legend has it that the Song emperor had lost his eldest son to smallpox, so he traveled deep into the forest of a high mountain and sought help from a reclusive nun. The woman was known as a holy healer, and she passed on the technique of variolation to save the ancient Chinese royal family.

Essential

Two to three percent of individuals receiving the variolation ended up dying from smallpox. The only reason this practice continued was because the chance of dying from smallpox caught "naturally" from another infected person was 15 to 20 percent.

The germ theory was unknown at the time when variolation was first invented, so the process of variolation was invented purely based on the intuition of a few observant people. However, the practice was not without risk. Virtually everyone variolated came down with a high fever. Getting variolated was a gamble.

Fact

Lady Mary Montagu was also a prominent pioneer in the feminist movement. Not only did she advocate for children's health, she played an important role in convincing the English royal family to accept variolation to protect them from smallpox.

The technique of variolation was passed on from ancient China to India and eventually made its way to the Middle East. The procedure was modified after hundreds of years, and the Turks practiced an alternative form of variolation. The Turkish procedure involved making a small cut on the skin and rubbing the drainage from a pustule of a person infected with smallpox into the small cut. Similar to the Chinese variolation process, the inoculated person would often get sick but almost always recovered with a lifelong immunity against smallpox.

Lady Mary Wortley Montagu was an English aristocrat who married a diplomat to Istanbul. She was famous for her extraordinary beauty and sharp wit, until her flawless facial features were tarnished by a bout with smallpox. Her brother also died from smallpox. She was the person credited for bringing the practice of variolation from the Middle East to Europe.

🅐 Alert

Variolation is a far riskier procedure than today's vaccination. In fact, it was so dangerous that it was outlawed in all of the American colonies except in the city of Philadelphia. Thomas Jefferson believed in the procedure, and he had to travel to the City of Brotherly Love to get variolated.

While living in Turkey with her husband, she witnessed the local Turks variolating each other to avoid getting the smallpox infection. She was impressed by the protective effect of variolation, and she had her five-year-old son and four-year-old daughter inoculated. Being a prominent figure in the political arena, she introduced the practice of variolation to the political elites back in Europe. When a smallpox epidemic swept through England, the royal family became anxious, but they were also hesitant to get variolated because it was such an unorthodox procedure. To reassure themselves that the procedure was safe enough, they offered prisoners facing the death sentence a chance at redemption if they volunteered to receive variolation. Six prisoners offered to be guinea pigs for this medical experiment, and they all survived the variolation procedure. In addition, they did not get the smallpox infection when they were intentionally exposed to victims of small-pox. After witnessing such success with variolation, the royal family was convinced and had their children variolated against smallpox. The royal family escaped the wrath of smallpox unscathed.

Ironically, the medical establishment at the time was the primary and most vocal opponent of variolation. It was an untested procedure, and it involved intentionally making healthy people sick. It was also well known that people died from variolation, and variolation was illegal in the American colonies. Only a few maverick doctors were brave enough to variolate people, and these doctors faced death threats from early vaccine opponents.

When variolation was first introduced during the smallpox epidemic of 1721 in Boston, it was viewed with skepticism and fear. Many in the Puritan town viewed the smallpox outbreak as divine judgment, and it would be heresy to thwart the will of God. People also feared the procedure, and with good reason, because the technique at the time—rubbing the pus from an infected person into a small cut on the arm or leg of a healthy individual—was indeed barbaric and crude. Finally, people had gotten extremely sick and even died from variolation, and the variolated person could transmit smallpox to other unvariolated people. There was good reason for people to hesitate about getting variolated.

While the controversy was brewing in the American colonies, Edward Jenner, an English physician, vastly reduced the side effects and danger of variolation by introducing the first modern vaccine. While working as an apprentice surgeon in rural England, he made the observation that while smallpox seemed to be rampant in the countryside, milkmaids generally were unaffected by this common infection. In fact, milkmaids were known for their uncanny fair complexion because their countenance was spared the scars of smallpox infections.

Dr. Jenner also realized that milkmaids were frequently afflicted with another condition called cowpox. This disease was uncommon in the general public, but it looked like a milder form of smallpox. In contrast with smallpox infection, cowpox infection did not leave its victim permanently scarred, and death was extremely rare. From these observations, Dr. Jenner hypothesized that by working closely with cows, milkmaids unintentionally became immune to smallpox infection by getting the cowpox infection first. He was also aware of the practice of variolation, and he subsequently derived his own technique of variolation.

Instead of using the pus or scab from a smallpox victim, he used material isolated from people infected with cowpox, a related infection that isn't nearly as deadly. When the body is exposed to cowpox, he surmised that the body then develops immunity against smallpox as well because the germ causing cowpox is so similar to smallpox. This practice is now known as vaccination, which is a significant improvement to variolation because the risks of serious side effects from smallpox vaccination are much smaller than smallpox variolation.

 Fact

George Washington initially balked at variolating his troops. After two major losses to the British troops, who were all variolated, General Washington started inoculating the American soldiers. The region of Quebec could have very well ended up as American territory today if the American troops were variolated earlier in the Revolutionary War.

When Dr. Jenner first proposed the new technique of vaccination, his research paper went largely unnoticed. In fact, many of his colleagues ridiculed him for coming up with such a ludicrous idea of employing "alternative" medicine that originated from the Orient and Middle East. Cartoonists lampooned him and the process of vaccination, drawing caricatures of vaccinated individuals as having horns and hooves like cows.

To convince the public, he successfully performed the procedure on an eight-year-old boy named James Phipps. The material was isolated from the blisters of a milkmaid who had caught cowpox. Following his vaccination, James escaped an outbreak of smallpox in his town completely unaffected while other children perished. After his proven success with the vaccine, Dr. Jenner vaccinated his own son with the cowpox vaccine.

Beginning of Mass Immunization

By the late 1800s, Jenner's smallpox vaccine was more or less accepted by the public. A hundred years of experience using the vaccine had shown that vaccination can be safe and effective, but only the privileged few could afford vaccination. Smallpox outbreaks still occurred because the majority of the population was not vaccinated.

Scientists at the turn of the century were beginning to understand that germs were responsible for infectious diseases. A renewed effort saw the invention of additional vaccines to fight rampant outbreaks of diphtheria and whooping cough. At the time, diphtheria wreaked havoc in the communities, and the only treatment available was using antitoxin to combat the poison released by this bacteria. The treatment was wrought with problems, even though it was quite effective in saving lives. The antitoxin was derived from horse serum. Consequently, many children who received the antitoxin serum developed severe and sometimes life-threatening allergic reactions. A better way was to prevent the infection in the first place rather than subject sick people to a dangerous treatment. As a result of this effort, the diphtheria vaccine was developed.

Shortly after the invention of the diphtheria vaccine, the tetanus vaccine became available, which was followed by the whooping cough vaccine. These vaccines were an important part of the war effort during World War II, and routine vaccination of soldiers played a major role in reducing casualties on the battlefield. The tetanus vaccine played an especially important role in reducing deaths from battle wounds. During World War I, the leading cause of death from combat was tetanus. Even a relatively minor cut could trigger this almost fatal infection. Compared to the millions that perished from tetanus during the First World War, less than a handful died from tetanus during the Second World War. The difference was the tetanus vaccine.

HISTORICAL TIMELINE FOR CHILDHOOD IMMUNIZATION:

- **1796** - first vaccine for smallpox (no longer used in children)
- **1924** - first vaccine for tetanus
- **1924** - first vaccine for diphtheria
- **1926** - first vaccine for pertussis (whooping cough)
- **1945** - first vaccine for influenza
- **1954** - first vaccine for polio (injected Salk vaccine)
- **1964** - first vaccine for measles
- **1967** - first vaccine for mumps
- **1970** - first vaccine for rubella
- **1974** - first vaccine for chickenpox
- **1977** - first vaccine for pneumonia (*Streptococcus pneumoniae*)
- **1978** - first vaccine for meningitis (*Neisseria meningitidis*)
- **1981** - first vaccine for hepatitis B
- **1985** - first vaccine for *Haemophilus influenzae* type b (Hib)
- **1992** - first vaccine for hepatitis A
- **1998** - first vaccine for rotavirus
- **2006** - first vaccine for the human papilloma virus

The 1970s and 1980s witnessed an explosion in the development of new vaccines. Vaccines against measles, mumps, and rubella (German measles) came around in the 1970s, and the meningitis and hepatitis B vaccines rolled out in the 1980s. The introduction of so many vaccines in such a short period of time triggered much controversy. While scientists were busy coming up with new vaccines, the public felt overwhelmed and a backlash against the medical community ensued. Even though it was not the first time community activists took up arms against vaccination, it would later prove to be one of the most vocal and formidable social movements of our time.

Real Benefits

It is true that no vaccine is 100 percent effective. But it is also true that smallpox has become extinct due to the successful worldwide vaccination program. Polio is fast becoming the second disease heading toward that fate. These two devastating infections would still be rampaging humanity, as they have done for thousands of years, if it weren't for the global effort at vaccination.

Many people question whether vaccination is the real reason for the improvement of public health and reduction in infection. Around the same time mass public vaccination was initiated, sanitation and nutrition also improved. While it is reasonable to say that other factors contributed to the improvement in the health of the general population around the turn of the century, it is more difficult to say that sanitation has improved drastically from the 1980s to the 1990s. This is the time frame when childhood deaths and retardation from meningitis were reduced from epidemic levels to near zero. This reduction in meningitis among children coincided with the introduction of two vaccines against meningitis.

The story of the Hib and pneumococcal vaccines is one of the major victories of modern science. Hib is a bacterium that used to cause more meningitis in children than any other bacteria, and the consequences of this dangerous brain infection were devastating. If your child managed to survive the brain infection (and many did not), she often became deaf or retarded because the infection had destroyed so much brain tissue. This infection used to be the most common cause of mental retardation in the United States.

Since its introduction in 1985, the Hib brain infection has become an extremely rare disease. This infection is so rare now that most doctors who finished their medical training since the 1990s have never seen a child with Hib meningitis.

Fortunately, vaccines do not have to work 100 percent of the time to save lives; in fact, none of the vaccines work well all the time. Much like seat belts and bystander CPR, vaccines save lives as long as they work most of the time. The concept of *herd immunity* is behind the success of community-wide vaccination programs.

✱ Essential

Herd immunity works both ways. It protects the whole group if the majority of people are vaccinated, protecting the few who are not. But if the majority of people are not immunized, even those who are vaccinated are at risk of becoming infected because vaccination does not offer 100 percent protection.

To understand herd immunity, imagine a group of drivers on the road. As long as the majority of the drivers follow traffic rules, the number of traffic accidents is limited. Even if a few reckless drivers maneuver their cars irresponsibly, the majority of the careful drivers could avoid accident by using defensive driving techniques. However, if the majority of the drivers become reckless, then it would be impossible for the minority careful drivers to avoid accidents.

Similarly, if the majority of children are vaccinated in a population, it would be very difficult for a germ to spread. Even if a few children come down with the infection, the germ cannot spread easily because most of the other children around the infected child are immunized. It is not impossible for an outbreak to occur, but the odds are against the germs.

On the other hand, if the majority of the children are not vaccinated, then the few who are would make very little difference in curbing the spread of infection. Most of the people that the germ comes in contact with are susceptible to the infection, so the germ can spread easily and quickly throughout the entire population. Even though the few who are vaccinated are less likely to get sick, a large proportion of the group will end up with the disease.

Real Risks

The path to the modern vaccination program was not without perils. In the early days of the smallpox vaccine, many children got sick and some died from contaminated vaccines. These complications were caused by the inoculation technique of the time. Sterilization was not utilized, and the needle used for the immunization was commonly contaminated with bacteria. Through the small puncture wound during the vaccination process, bacteria can gain entrance into the skin and cause infection. Some of these infections led to fatalities.

Alert

In 1942, the military accidentally infected more than 300,000 soldiers with hepatitis B when they received contaminated yellow fever vaccines. Fifty-one thousand military personnel were hospitalized for hepatitis, and up to 100 people died from liver cancer resulting from the hepatitis B infection.

When the killed polio vaccine was first introduced in 1954, vaccine manufacturers lacked experience in the vaccine production process. Strict protocols were not followed, and government oversight was lax. One of the early vaccine producers released vaccines contaminated with live polio virus, and hundreds of children became paralyzed by the vaccine. A few died. Following this fiasco, regulations were quickly instituted, but the damage was done. The public's trust in vaccination was deeply shaken. The vaccine manufacturer responsible for the accident was the now defunct Cutter Laboratories, and the infamous event was known as the Cutter incident.

In 1947, 6 million people in New York were vaccinated against smallpox because a traveler had contracted the infection and brought it back to Manhattan. He subsequently died from smallpox, and two more deaths followed. Panic spread through the city and demand quickly outstripped the existing vaccine supply. A vaccine shortage ensued. (It was later determined that all three victims were in close contact, and a citywide outbreak would never occur.) By the time an outbreak was ruled out, millions of people had already received the vaccine unnecessarily. Many of those people experienced mild to moderate side effects from the vaccine.

These mistakes serve as a reminder that vaccines are powerful tools, and they can be double-edged swords. Used improperly, they can cause great bodily harm and become a tremendous public health burden. Close monitoring of vaccine production and storage is paramount to a successful and safe vaccine program.

The Evolution of the Modern Immunization

Today's vaccines are definitely not your parents' vaccines. In the past forty years, many new vaccines have been invented and many old ones have been retired. Doctors are always weighing the risks and benefits of each vaccine to come up with new recommendations. The immunization schedule is modified annually, and sometimes more frequently than that. New infections come and old infections go, so the risk of getting an infection is always changing. Many factors play into the changing landscape, including the frequent use of antibiotics, immigration, and an ever-increasing number of people who choose not to be vaccinated.

Unlike some of the earlier vaccines, many of the newer vaccines are designed not to prevent deaths but to decrease suffering and hospitalization. For example, chickenpox is not usually a fatal infection, and most children who get chickenpox recover completely. However, chickenpox is responsible for school absenteeism, and it does cause fever, a bad itchy rash, and some discomfort. In rare circumstances, chickenpox can cause a serious skin infection that may require amputation of a part of an arm or leg to keep the infection from spreading. So when the chickenpox vaccine was developed, it wasn't aimed at saving lives for the most part, but it was made available to prevent so many children from missing school and being very uncomfortable.

✅ Fact

More than 100,000 children end up in the hospital each year due to diarrhea, and about 50,000 children stay in the hospital for many days to receive intravenous fluid due to severe dehydration. Less than 100 children die from this infection each year in the United States, so rotavirus infection is rarely fatal.

Another example of a new vaccine is the rotavirus vaccine. Similar to chickenpox, most children in developed countries do not die from rotavirus. Rotavirus causes very bad diarrhea, and babies are especially susceptible to this infection. The diarrhea is extremely watery and can happen more than twenty times a day. The rotavirus vaccine was developed to help babies stay healthy and reduce the burden for parents in taking care of their sick children.

Some parents question the necessity of these newer vaccines because these vaccines are not designed to prevent fatal illnesses. Diaper rashes, regardless of how severe, are not fatal illnesses either. Whether you need to do anything to prevent and treat diaper rash is a personal choice also.

In addition to the introduction of new vaccines, there are some older vaccines that are no longer given to children because the infections they are designed to prevent are so rare now. In 1971 the smallpox vaccine was retired because smallpox is technically extinct. Starting in 2000, American children no longer receive the oral polio vaccine because polio has become an extremely rare condition in the United States. Doctors will continue to consider retiring additional vaccines when the infections they help to prevent become so rare that it no longer make sense to continue vaccination against them.

The childhood immunization schedule has changed every single year since 2000. Consult your pediatrician for the most up-to-date immunization schedule for your child.

The Informed Parent Movement

In the past, most parents accepted standardized childhood immunization as a rite of passage. In the 1970s, most parents did not question the necessity of vaccination and were happy to have their children vaccinated. In fact, most parents did not even realize that a choice existed for parents to decline vaccination. The childhood immunization program was perceived as a public mandate, and it was one's civic duty to protect children and the community from infectious diseases.

Today's parents play a much more active role in making medical decisions for their children. After all, you are the most trusted advocate for your child. In the past, parents relied on their trust in the medical profession in delivering the best preventative and curative options, but today's parents are much savvier. The relationship between the parents and the pediatrician has evolved into a collaborative effort that focuses on the best interest of the children.

Unfortunately, a rift has recently opened in this collaboration. Many parents no longer trust the medical establishment or the scientific community. They view doctors as either greedy or ignorant pawns of the pharmaceutical industry and vaccination as carried out not to protect children but to intentionally harm babies so that the medical community can profit from their suffering.

Many factors have contributed to this rift, including the rising tide of autism, inability of parents to have their own doctors, and the easy access to the Internet and inaccurate or obsolete information. Since parents think they can no longer trust their doctors to provide reliable information, they have no choice but to become their own advocate and form their own coalitions to exchange ideas and information. This certainly is a new and empowering experience for many parents.

🔔 Alert

Many websites are designed to sell books or herbal supplements, and they will write anything to attract the attention of parents. If the website prominently features advertisements for any product (books, supplements, appointments), be very wary of the information it presents.

However, many online communities formed by parents do not have any input from doctors or scientists. Doctors trained in conventional medicine rarely interact with these new parental online communities. What makes matters worse is that these communities often face an angry response from the medical community, therefore further widening the existing gap. Besides the angry exchange of words, there is little actual communication between the parents and doctors in these settings. What is sorely needed is for both sides to stop lashing out at each other and listen to each other's perspective to sort out the misunderstanding. Many medical professionals are often impatient and unwilling to hear what the parents have to say. It's easy to understand why so many parents turn to these resources instead of their doctors for information because at least they can get a sympathetic ear when communicating with other parents.

If you read information on vaccines on the Internet, you should always keep in mind that there is no way to tell who is writing the information and whether they have ulterior motives for the information. The only information that is trustworthy is from a doctor with whom you have developed an ongoing relationship. If your doctor is unwilling or unable to spend the time to answer your questions, it is time to look for a new doctor for your child.

CHAPTER 2

How Do Vaccines Work?

T here is a lot of inaccurate information on how vaccines work. Some people think that vaccines weaken the body and make people more vulnerable to getting sick from other infections. Others believe that vaccines cause controlled infections when they immunize individuals. Even though there is a grain of truth in some of these ideas, the amount of misinformation is staggering. The goal of this chapter is to clear up the misconceptions and provide an accurate overview for everyone to understand.

The Human Immune System

Before embarking on a discussion about vaccines, you must first understand the role of the immune system. The immune system is your body's defense against germs. You can think of it as the armed forces for the body. It is essential for survival, since germs are ubiquitous and they constantly besiege the body, finding any opportunity for an invasion. Every day represents a constant battle between your body's immune system and germs.

To illustrate the importance of the immune system, just look at what happens when the immune system is absent or weakened. Cancer patients who are undergoing chemotherapy and patients with AIDS (acquired immune deficiency syndrome) have severely weakened immune systems. Their immune systems are under siege either from the underlying illness (cancer, AIDS) or from the actual treatment for their condition (chemotherapy). They are vulnerable to a host of infections that most people never have to worry about. These individuals with devastated immune systems must be constantly on guard with what they eat, where they can go, and who is around them. They must take all these precautions to compensate for their lack of defenses against invading germs.

Germs and You

Most people assume that if an object or surface appears clean it is free of germs. This is far from the truth. Unless an object exists under sterile conditions (that is, no dust, never been touched by anyone or anything), it is probably contaminated with bacteria. Dust particles are actually common carriers of bacteria, including the tetanus bacteria and bacteria that cause infant botulism.

Furthermore, the human body is coinhabited by bacteria. There are bacteria that live on your skin, inside your mouth and nose, and in your intestinal tract. Thanks to the constant vigilance of your immune system, they are held in check. In fact, your body most likely reaps some benefit from these bacteria.

For example, the bacteria that live on the skin protect you from fungal infections (such as ringworms). These bacteria are normally harmless, and by covering the skin, they prevent fungus from squatting on the same skin surface. This is the reason why you are more likely to get yeast infections when you take antibiotics. The antibiotics eradicate the bad germs, but they also take out the "good" germs covering your skin. The absence of these "good" germs allows the fungus to establish on the skin and spread.

In addition, the bacteria inhabiting your gut provide essential vitamin K for your body. When the bacteria ferment food material inside your intestine, they create vitamin K as a byproduct. Since vitamin K is not stored in large quantity in the body, the existence of these bacteria in your gut is not only beneficial but also essential. Vitamin K is necessary in allowing your blood to clot in case there is an injury.

 Fact

Newborn babies are prone to vitamin K deficiency partly because their intestines have not yet been colonized by bacteria, so they do not get the additional vitamin K produced by these beneficial bacteria normally found in an adult intestine. This is the rationale behind giving all newborn babies a vitamin K injection.

Even though these bacteria are helpful, they can cause dangerous infections for individuals with weakened immune systems. Premature babies have inadequate defenses because they are born too soon, so even these relatively benign germs that are harmless to everyone else can lead to life-threatening infections in these small babies. This further illustrates the importance of the immune system.

Essential

The immune system's memory does not work all the time. With certain types of germs, the immune system is unable to remember a previous infection and keep a record of it. An example for this is the Hib bacterium. Even after a serious infection caused by Hib, a baby's immune system does not remember the attack.

Most germs you hear about are not so kind as the ones just described. Not only won't they provide good vitamins for the body, they invade the body and wreak havoc on the normal functioning of the body. What makes the matter worse is that they are just as omnipresent as the good germs. The only chance that humanity has any hope of surviving in this germ-filled world is because of the diligent immune system.

The Defense Archive

In addition to being constantly vigilant, your immune system has another unique characteristic. It has the ability to keep track of germs that it has encountered in the past. In other words, germs that have invaded the body before are blacklisted by the immune system. The next time the same germ attempts to sneak into your body, your immune defense can recognize the old foe and eradicate it quickly.

This is an extremely useful characteristic of the immune system because it allows the body to gradually evolve over time and adapt to the most common germs. This way, the immune system doesn't need to mount a new attack each time it encounters germs, which allows your body to function much more efficiently and react more quickly in case of an infection. The invention of immunization takes advantage of this "memory" aspect of your immune system.

The Germ Police

How do vaccines take advantage of the memory of the immune system? Normally the immune system is alerted when the body detects the presence of a particular type of germ, and a biological profile of the germ is recorded as part of the immune system's archive. A useful analogy would be to compare this vast immune archive of germs to a police department's archive of criminals. Any criminal who was arrested also gets tracked by the police department. Similarly, the immune system creates a new record of a particular germ when it invades the body for the first time.

Of course, this means that no criminal record is made in the archive until a crime has been committed. This means that potential victims have already suffered by the time a criminal record is created.

But what if the police could capture a criminal before the crime has been committed? They would need detailed profiles of all criminals or would-be criminals.

Immunization does just that. It provides your immune system with detailed profiles of bad germs before they invade your body. It is like giving your immune system a heads-up before any germ attempts to invade. This is accomplished several ways. One way to provide identification of germs is by having a detailed and unique description of the germ targeted. Another way is to have the actual dead germs presented to the intelligence headquarters. Finally, live but severely weakened germs can be utilized to extract detailed intelligence for your defense system.

Dead or Alive

Vaccines can be divided into two major categories. Most vaccines are derived from parts of dead germs or the whole dead germs, but some vaccines actually contain live germs. They are made differently because some germs cannot trigger the alarm in your immune system once they are killed, so they must be presented to your immune system alive.

Before you start to get queasy from the thought of having live germs injected into your body, keep in mind that there are already live germs living inside your body. In addition, when you eat a plate of salad, you are in fact ingesting live plants. And if you are not a strict vegetarian, you are consuming animal carcasses every time you bite into a steak or a chicken drumstick. It sounds gross when you think about it, but the reality is that having other life forms in your body is neither unusual nor unnatural.

Vaccines Derived from Parts of Germs

Many vaccines are made from parts of germs. These vaccines cannot cause an infection because a single body part of a germ is not enough to allow the germ to spread in the body or cause any illness. Think of these vaccines as the physical characteristics of a terrorist for the police file, such as a tattoo or dental record. The police can safely keep this information in their headquarters without fearing the information causing a threat to security. The list of vaccines that are made from germ parts include vaccines against hepatitis A, hepatitis B, *Haemophilus influenza* type B, pneumococcus, and certain flu vaccines.

Vaccines Derived from Toxins

A few vaccines are designed from poisons created by germs. These vaccines work by alerting the body's defense to the toxin released by germs, giving the immune system a head start in getting rid of these poisonous chemicals. You can think of these types of vaccines as blueprints to the germ's weapons. Once again, these "blueprints" can be safely stored in police headquarters without compromising the security of the complex. A weapon is quite harmless unless it falls into the wrong hands. Inside the body, these modified toxins cannot be activated by anything, so they can only trigger the immune system and do not cause any problem. Examples of this type of vaccine include the tetanus and diphtheria vaccines.

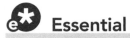 **Essential**

Unlike most other vaccines, the flu vaccine exists in two forms. There is a version of the flu vaccine that contains killed flu virus. This form comes in an injectable vaccine. There is another type of flu vaccine that is sprayed up the nose. The nasal spray flu vaccine contains actual live flu virus.

Vaccines Derived from Dead Germs

Some vaccines are produced from killed germs. These vaccines work by providing the immune system with a complete physical description of these germs, so when these germs attempt to invade the body, the body's defense will recognize them immediately and thwart their invasion. These vaccines cannot cause a real infection in the person receiving the vaccine because dead germs are unable to carry out their bad deeds. Vaccines that use this mechanism include polio, rabies, anthrax, typhoid, Japanese encephalitis, cholera, and most flu vaccines.

Vaccines Derived from Live Germs

Some people consider these types of vaccines the most dangerous because they are made from live germs. However, the germs in these vaccines are severely weakened. Nevertheless, they can cause a mild infection in the person receiving the vaccine. You can compare these types of vaccines to the police holding terrorists in custody. They do pose a security risk to the defense system, but they can yield even more valuable intelligence than a killed enemy because they can be interrogated by the body's immune system. If these bad guys escape from custody, your body may experience a very weak but real attack by these germs. The good news is that the mild case of the infection is never dangerous to a healthy person. Nevertheless, people with severely weakened immune systems should generally avoid getting live vaccines. Vaccines that fall under this description include measles, mumps, rubella (German measles), chickenpox, yellow fever, tuberculosis, and certain flu vaccines (the nasal spray flu vaccine, tradename FluMist).

How Well Do Vaccines Work?

One of the main arguments from vaccine opponents is that vaccines do not work. The fact is that there is no vaccine that can protect its recipient 100 percent of the time. It is entirely possible to receive a vaccine and still become infected from the germ that the vaccine is designed to protect. However, all vaccines do work most of the time. Keep in mind, however, that there are very few things in life that work perfectly all the time. Your car, your computer, and even your body will fail at one time or another, but you do not stop driving your car just because there is a possibility that it might malfunction.

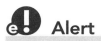 **Alert**

The chickenpox vaccine does not offer 100 percent protection to all of its recipients, either. Many children who have received the vaccine still got chickenpox, although the symptoms are much milder. This is the reason why doctors now recommend a booster chickenpox vaccine so that the shots can better protect your child.

Scientists and doctors know that certain vaccines work better than others. For example, vaccines against tetanus, polio, and smallpox work extremely well. These vaccines protect their recipients more than 99 percent of the time if they are exposed to these germs. On the other hand, it is well known to physicians and many patients that some vaccines do not always protect people from getting the infection. The flu vaccine is a good example. Even in communities where most of the members are vaccinated, outbreaks of flu can still occur in the winter.

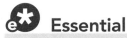 **Essential**

This differential in immune response is also seen in a scenario not involving vaccines. Most of you are aware that once a person recovers from the chickenpox he or she is immune for life. However, a small percentage of individuals may get chickenpox again for the second time.

Vaccines can fail for a number of reasons. Some people's immune systems are simply not as responsive to immunization as others. In addition, some people's response to the immunization fades more rapidly than others. In other words, these people's immune systems do not keep the record against germs as long as the majority of the population. For these individuals, the vaccines work temporarily, but the protection derived from vaccination wanes over time.

To put the effectiveness of vaccines in perspective, compare immunization to the use of seat belts. Wearing a seat belt doesn't give you the ability to cheat death. Although seat belt usage offers some degree of protection against serious injuries and death, it doesn't give you the license to drive recklessly. Even though seat belts do not always protect you from injuries in an accident, it doesn't mean that you should stop wearing one.

Limitations of Vaccines

Even with the plethora of vaccines, it is obvious that there are still many infections that can afflict you and your children. Not every disease can be prevented with a vaccine. HIV is an example where the vaccine development effort has stalled and scientists have failed to come up with a working vaccine despite decades of research (see Chapter 20 for a more detailed discussion on the HIV vaccine). As mentioned before, no vaccine works 100 percent of the time. Furthermore, the immunity generated after vaccination wanes after long period of time.

How long do vaccines work? This is a tricky question, because each person's immune system reacts to even the same vaccine differently. Going back to the police department analogy, the record keeping of the immune system is not perfect. After a long time (five to ten years, perhaps), the immune system's record on each particular germ becomes faded and outdated. Just as the police's profile of criminals needs to be updated on a regular basis to keep it relevant because the criminal could have been captured, deceased, or moved to a different location, the immune system needs a reminder every now and then to keep the relevant information on germs up-to-date.

The fact that the immune system's germ archive needs regular updates is the rationale behind booster shots. Not all vaccines require booster shots, but many do. Those vaccines that do not require lifelong boosting include vaccines against hepatitis B, hepatitis A, rotavirus, pneumococcus, and Hib. There are two reasons why these vaccines do not require additional booster after completing the initial series. For hepatitis A and B, the immune system's memory after the initial injections is quite long-lasting. Evidence shows that the vaccines remain effective between fifteen to twenty years after the completion of the series of vaccines. The effect may last longer, but the evidence is unavailable at this time because these vaccines have not been around for that long yet.

🔴 Alert

While it is true that the "memory" of germs lasts longer after a child gets an infection naturally than from immunization, even natural immunity wanes over a period of time. Immunity against RSV, a common childhood respiratory infection, is incomplete at best. Babies often get RSV infection year after year.

With the vaccines for rotavirus, pneumococcal, and Hib infections, booster vaccines are not routinely recommended because infections caused by these two bacteria pose very little threat to anyone older than five years of age. It would not matter much if older children get sick from these infections because the immune system is generally stronger for older children and adults.

Other vaccines, including shots for tetanus, whooping cough, measles, mumps, rubella, and polio, require booster injections to update the immune system's record on these germs. The vaccines for tetanus and whooping cough are especially unique because a regular booster is needed every ten years, even into adulthood. You are never too old to get the tetanus booster vaccine.

The bottom line is that very few vaccines can protect a person indefinitely. But the same is true for an infection that occurs naturally. If your child survived a whooping cough infection, it is still possible to get whooping cough again later on in life. The immunity after a whooping cough infection lasts four to twenty years after the infection. It does not protect your child forever. The same thing goes for chickenpox. It is definitely possible to get chickenpox twice, or even three times.

✅ Fact

The pneumococcus bacterium can cause serious problems in elderly individuals, but a different type of pneumococcal vaccine is recommended for older people (the pneumococcal polysaccharide vaccine). Only children receive the conjugate pneumococcal vaccine. See Chapter 11 for a detailed discussion on the pneumococcal vaccine.

The immune system's record of germs does not work perfectly, and the immune system's memory does not last a lifetime. This is one of the reasons why your child can get sick from cold and stomach viruses year after year, regardless of how many times he has already gotten sick before.

CHAPTER 3

Vaccine Reactions

No one would deny the fact that vaccination can trigger some unwanted reactions. While most of these reactions are mild and transient, some reactions can be devastating. It is extremely important for parents to understand these reactions and know what to do about them if they occur. Recognizing these reactions and how often they happen is indispensable for making the right decision for your child.

Common Reactions

While everyone's attention tends to focus on the serious and long-lasting side effects of vaccines, you must not overlook the relatively minor reactions that are commonly associated with vaccination. Even though these reactions are mild and tend to go away on their own, they can nevertheless be the source of parental stress and anxiety. This section will explore these reactions and discuss ways to ameliorate them.

Fever

Most parents know that children can develop a fever after routine vaccination, but you may not know just how often a fever can occur and when to call the doctor about a fever. Not all vaccines cause fever after administration, but most can. Even among the vaccines that may trigger a fever, only about 10–20 percent of children will develop a fever after these vaccines. So even though fever is a common postvaccination reaction, it does not happen more than half of the time. It is very likely that your child may be completely fine after receiving her vaccination.

 Fact

The following vaccines only cause fever in rare circumstances: the HPV vaccine, the hepatitis A vaccine, the meningococcal vaccine, and the polio vaccine. These vaccines differ from most other vaccines because they do not trigger a fever in most cases.

Fever is your body's alarm system. When the immune system goes into high-alert mode, it sends a signal to the body, and the part of your brain that controls body temperature elevates the set temperature for the entire body and you develop a fever.

In children, fevers usually happen because there is an infection. In case of vaccination, there is no "real" infection going on, but the immune system can go into a high-alert mode because it may perceive that there is a germ invasion going on. Think of the fever triggered by vaccination as the body's defense system having a mock drill in preparation for a germ invasion. While there is no threat, the defenses are up and the body learns how to fight off a real infection if it were to occur in the future.

The technical definition of a fever is when your child's temperature rises above 100.3°F (38° Celsius). While the exact body temperature is important when determining the presence of a fever, how the temperature is taken and the circumstances when the temperature is taken are equally important.

There are several types of thermometers and several ways you can take the temperature of your child. If your baby is less than three months old, the best and most reliable way of taking the temperature is through a digital rectal thermometer. However, this method of measuring body temperature can be slightly uncomfortable for the baby, and some parents may feel uneasy with the procedure.

🔔 Alert

The ear thermometer, or the tympanic thermometer, scans the body temperature by reading the infrared radiation from the body. While it is quick and easy to take the temperature, the temperature reading from this type of thermometer is inaccurate and unreliable, especially if your child is less than six months of age.

The next best way to measure the temperature is in the mouth, but this is only feasible for older children who will not try to eat the thermometer when you put it inside the mouth. Inserting the thermometer under the armpit (also called the axillary temperature) is a good compromise between ease of taking the temperature and accuracy. While the body temperature measured in the armpit tends to be somewhat lower than the actual rectal temperature, it is close enough for the parents to get an idea of the body temperature. Even though many thermometer instructions recommend adding a degree or two to an axillary temperature, doing so may overestimate the actual temperature and cause a false alarm for fever.

Finally, you need to take your child's surroundings into consideration when interpreting a high temperature. If your child is bundled up in several thick layers of wooly blanket on a hot summer afternoon, the body temperature can rise significantly. This doesn't necessarily mean that your child has a fever. If the recorded temperature is high and your baby may be too hot from overbundling, unwrap the baby for ten minutes and recheck the temperature. If the temperature continues to be high, then a real fever may be present.

While the fever triggered by vaccination is not dangerous, it can still be alarming to parents and uncomfortable for the child. A vaccine-induced fever is usually very short lasting. Such fever rarely lasts for more than two days, and three days of fever after immunization is quite unexpected.

ⓔ✱ Essential

If your child has a fever for more than two days after vaccination, you should take him to the doctor's office and have him checked out for other causes of the fever. Your doctor may not elect to do any blood tests or x-rays at that time, depending on your child's physical examination in the office.

What if the fever is very high after vaccination? Is that a cause for concern? Not necessarily. First of all, a high fever is when the body's temperature rises above 102°F. Two to five percent of children may develop a fever that high after vaccination, so it would not be too unusual. However, if the temperature goes higher than 104°F after vaccination, most doctors would consider doing some evaluation (such as blood tests) to ensure that there is nothing else that could be causing the high fever. Whenever you are uncertain about any vaccine reaction, give your doctor a call.

Since most children will not develop a fever after vaccination, routine administration of over-the-counter fever reducers (acetaminophen, ibuprofen) beforehand is generally not recommended. Giving every child medication to prevent a minority with fever is unnecessary at best and possibly harmful at times. Consult your doctor about the dosage of fever reducer if you plan to use these medications.

Besides using fever-reducing medications, you may also utilize other cooling measures for postvaccination fever. You can increase the fluid intake for your child, and you can soak a towel with room-temperature water and drape the wet towel over your child's bare shoulder. Remember, fever after vaccination is not dangerous. Measures to reduce the temperature are primarily to make your child more comfortable and reduce your own anxiety.

 Alert

> If you elect to use a fever reducer to treat your child's fever, use acetaminophen (Tylenol). You may use ibuprofen (Motrin) if your child is older than six months of age. Avoid using aspirin for any child under all circumstances because aspirin can cause a fatal reaction in children called Reye's syndrome.

Whether the fever is triggered by the vaccine or caused by a real infection, an elevated body temperature itself is never dangerous for your child. There is a popular belief that if the temperature gets too high it can cause permanent brain damage. This is never the case. No matter how high the fever goes, it will not cause harm to your child. The only exception to this rule is if your child's temperature is high because the surrounding environment does not allow the body to dissipate heat. If the body gets trapped in a very hot environment (hot tub, the desert) and cannot lower the temperature by sweating, the resulting high body temperature can lead to heat stroke, which can be life threatening. Generally speaking, body temperature never exceeds more than 106°F, unless the outside environment is the reason for the elevated temperature.

Swelling

The skin where the injection was given can sometimes swell up after vaccination. This does not happen with the majority of injections, but it can occur up to 20 percent of the time with some vaccines. Even though it is relatively common, the good news is that the degree of swelling is not usually related to the amount of pain. It is quite common for children to have an extremely large swelling but have absolutely no pain in the swollen area.

The best thing to do for the swelling is apply a cool washcloth over the swollen area. You can also use ibuprofen to reduce the swelling, but avoid using aspirin in children. A heating pad is generally not recommended because it tends to worsen the swelling.

ⓔ✱ Essential

If the swelling covers a large area of the body or if the swelling is accompanied with significant pain or tenderness, contact the doctor immediately. Swelling after vaccination is usually painless or minimally painful. A very painful reaction is likely the result of poor vaccination technique.

Irritability

This can vary anywhere from a mild fussiness to full-blown nonstop screaming for hours on end. Obviously, the difference between the degrees of severity of the reaction matters a great deal. Fortunately, the inconsolable crying that lasts more than three hours is an uncommon reaction that is only associated with the DTaP vaccine. Most children do not cry excessively after injections, and the crying rarely lasts for more than ten minutes. If the crying continues for more than an hour, call your doctor.

For mild, short-lasting irritability, you can calm your child by cradling her or rocking her in your arms. If your child wants to sleep, it is perfectly safe for her to take an early nap. Even though acetaminophen (Tylenol) has not been shown to be effective in reducing this irritability, it's a relatively safe remedy and you can administer it if you wish.

Drowsiness

Your baby may become sleepier after getting vaccinated. He may take a longer nap than usual or actually sleep through the night following immunization. This reaction is not dangerous, and most parents actually welcome the rare respite after not being able to sleep eight hours straight for months.

This reaction is harmless and does not require any treatment. Your baby will usually return to his regular sleeping routine a day or two after the immunization. Enjoy the long naps while you can.

Easing the Pain

This is an often overlooked topic in the discussion about vaccination. Most parents accept the pain associated with shots because it is short lasting and does not appear to have any permanent effect on babies. Some may even go as far as claiming that these acute pain episodes build character for their children.

Actually, it's not as simple as it seems. Some doctors have found that the short-lasting pain from injection and blood draws seems to influence the perception of pain in babies later on in life. Babies who have undergone a large number of poking seem to become more sensitive to pain in the future.

If this is surprising to you, you are not alone. Most doctors and nurses do not believe that a quick injection can have long-term effects. Consequently, most children (especially babies) do not receive any pain control prior to painful procedures.

Now that you know children can experience lasting effects after receiving injections, what can you do to help your child for a painful injection? Oral pain medications, including acetaminophen (Tylenol) or ibuprofen (Motrin), typically work poorly for sudden, sharp pain. These medications work wonderfully for a headache or dull ear pain, but they do not do much to alleviate acute pain.

There are several ways that you can help to reduce the pain your child feels. During the injection, give your baby a pacifier dipped in sugar water. You can also request a prescription for a topical pain-relieving cream from your doctor in advance and apply it to the injection site on the skin an hour prior to vaccination.

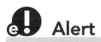 **Alert**

Be cautious with giving your baby store-bought herbal remedies. Some herbal remedies for colic and pain relief contain honey or sweetener derived from natural plants. These plant-based tinctures may be contaminated with the spores that can cause infant botulism. If the spores get inside your baby, she can become paralyzed and potentially die.

Finally, don't underestimate the power of distraction. You probably use this technique all the time at home to divert the attention of your child and stop her from playing with something dirty or dangerous. Distraction works equally well for a painful procedure.

It may be helpful if you ask your child to recall a pleasant experience, like visiting an amusement park or spending the weekend with grandparents. Alternatively, you can bring her favorite toy from home to have some degree of familiarity at the doctor's office. Many pediatric offices also give out cartoon stickers or small toys to children prior to injections.

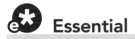 **Essential**

A stuffed animal, a favorite toy or book, or even the hand of a caregiver can provide great comfort for a child during a painful procedure. Don't be afraid to be creative and request the cooperation of the nurse or doctor who is giving the injection.

Another tried and true technique in reducing the pain sensation during an injection is asking your child to "blow out the candle." You can hold a small piece of paper and ask him to blow it away, or you can simply hold out your finger and pretend it's a candle. Ask your child to blow it out during an injection. While he exerts energy and focuses on your finger, he feels the painful sensation a lot less.

Calming your child not only has the benefit of alleviating pain, but it also increases the chance that the injection is given properly. A squirming and crying child is more likely to disrupt the technique and cause an accidental needle injury. A comfortable child can make the job easier for the person giving the injection, and that should be enough incentive for the care provider to ease your child's pain.

Serious Side Effects

Aside from the brief, relatively mild reactions that are attributable to vaccines, there are some rare but very serious reactions after vaccination. One of the most dangerous reactions is a whole-body allergic reaction called *anaphylaxis*. Another reaction is a devastating neurological condition called Guillain Barré Syndrome.

Anaphylaxis

Anaphylaxis occurs when the body reacts to an ingredient in the vaccine and causes the liquid part of the blood to leak out of the blood vessels and into the tissues. With this massive leaking of bodily fluid, the lungs fill with fluid and the throat swells shut, causing asphyxiation. This reaction could potentially occur with any vaccine. It is impossible to know when it might happen or who may have the reaction. The only saving grace is that this type of reaction is quite rare—about a one in a million occurrence.

On the other hand, this exact same reaction could occur with any food. A severe food allergy could just as easily trigger anaphylaxis. So every time you introduce a new food to your child, the potential for death is ever present. Peanut products and seafood are especially prone to causing such reaction, and this is the reason why pediatricians and dieticians recommend postponing the introduction of these foods until your child is at least three years old.

⊕ Alert

If your child has a severe allergic reaction (anaphylaxis) to chicken eggs, she should not receive the flu vaccine or the yellow fever vaccine. The MMR vaccine is made from chicken cells, and it contains a very small amount of egg protein. Anaphylactic reaction is very unlikely for people with egg allergy.

Guillain Barré Syndrome

Another serious reaction that can occur after certain vaccinations is Guillain Barré Syndrome. Guillain Barré Syndrome is a neurological condition that results from the immune system attacking one's own nervous system. Guillain Barré Syndrome frequently leads to temporary paralysis of the body because the immune system targets the nerves in the spinal cord that controls movement. You may also lose sensation of your arm and legs because the nerves responsible for feelings can also become affected.

Guillain Barré Syndrome is not common. It affects 1 in 100,000 people in the United States each year. Most cases of Guillain Barré Syndrome are triggered by infections. When germs invade your body, your immune system mounts a counterattack to fend off the invaders. This is usually a good thing, except when your body's immune system becomes overzealous and starts attacking your own body after the germ invasion has been fended off. If the immune system attacks the nerves in the spinal cord, Guillain Barré Syndrome may happen.

Two vaccines have been shown to trigger Guillain Barré Syndrome in humans—the flu vaccine and the meningococcal conjugate vaccine (trade name Menactra). Multiple scientific studies have shown that the flu vaccine can increase slightly the risk of developing Guillain Barré Syndrome. A few researchers have found that the meningococcal vaccine can trigger a similar reaction. However, the actual risk of developing paralysis from these two vaccines is quite small—about one in a million.

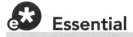 **Essential**

Guillain Barré Syndrome can be treated with immune-modifying medications. These treatment modalities do not always work, but they have been shown to improve strength and shorten the duration of the illness in some patients.

Fortunately, more than 70 percent of the people affected by Guillain Barré Syndrome fully recover, although the road to complete recovery is slow. It may take weeks to months to regain full use of the extremities. Some may be left with permanent disabilities.

Weighing the Risks

Now that you know vaccines can indeed cause serious and even fatal reactions, why are these vaccines still recommended by doctors? It's all about balancing the risks and benefits of vaccines.

While dangerous vaccine reactions are very real, so are the risks of life-threatening complications from infections. The flu strikes one in five people in the United States during many winter outbreaks, and about 36,000 people die from the flu each year in this country alone. Young babies and older adults are most vulnerable to the infection, and they are more likely to suffer life-threatening complications from the flu. Furthermore, these grim statistics only describe a typical flu season. During a flu pandemic, when a particular aggressive strain of the flu virus circulates around the globe, even more devastation may result.

As for the meningococcal vaccine, there is a one in a million chance of it triggering Guillain Barré Syndrome. The meningococcal infection occurs in 1 out of 100,000 individuals, but the risk is several times higher among college students living in dormitories. About 10 percent of people with the infection die from it. Even though there is antibiotic treatment for the meningococcal infection, the infection spreads through the body so rapidly that it is often too late by the time the diagnosis is made and treatment instituted.

✅ Fact

During the 1918 flu pandemic, 25 million people died from the flu within six months. As a comparison, it took AIDS twenty-five years to kill 25 million people, and 25 million soldiers lost their lives during the entire seven years of World War II.

When you crunch the numbers, you may realize that the chance of developing Guillain Barré Syndrome from the meningococcal vaccine and the chance of dying from meningococcal infection is about equal for noncollege students. However, keep in mind that most people with Guillain Barré Syndrome do not die from it, and permanent disability occurs in 15 percent of them. So even if you are not a college student living in a dormitory (for whom the chance of infection is much higher), you are still better off getting the vaccine. It is arguably better to suffer paralysis for a few months than to be dead. The beneficial odds for the vaccine are even better if you ever plan to go to college and stay in the dorms.

Everything you do involves risk, so the trick is how to play the odds and have them in your favor as frequently as possible.

Tracking Vaccine Reactions

A national registry has been set up to facilitate reporting and tracking all side effects potentially caused by vaccines. The Vaccine Adverse Event Reporting System (VAERS) is a centralized organization that analyzes all potential vaccine reactions. Anyone, including doctors and parents, can submit a report of a possible vaccine side effect directly to the national database.

As a parent, how can you be sure that the organization actually carries out its mission? How can you trust that the people analyzing the data do not have any conflict of interests and allow harmful vaccines to stay on the market?

To be sure, the system has already worked in the past. In 1998, when the first rotavirus vaccine was licensed for wide release, a rare but potentially fatal reaction was detected less than a year after the vaccine was in use. The VAERS quickly identified this possible side effect, and the RotaShield vaccine was immediately taken off the market. Even though the risk of experiencing this serious side effect was very small (less than 1 in 10,000), doctors and pharmaceutical companies did not hesitate to stop this vaccine. Not only do doctors want to avoid harming their patients, vaccine manufacturers certainly do not welcome any possible lawsuits resulting from an identifiable side effect. For a more detailed discussion on the rotavirus vaccine, read Chapter 12. To learn how you can report a possible vaccine-related side effect, refer to Appendix C.

CHAPTER 4

Vaccine Safety

A midst the controversy revolving around vaccines, what parents are most concerned about is the safety of vaccines. There is good reason to be worried, because immunization has caused severe reactions and sometimes permanent disabilities. Children have died as a result of getting vaccinated. This chapter is devoted to sort through and present the facts on vaccine safety.

Risk of Immunization

The risk of immunization is real; it was just made more apparent by the modern antivaccine movement. The public has always been skeptical of vaccines, but the wide availability of media and fast, global communication makes it easier for the word to get around and keep parents informed.

Vaccine Roulette

In 1982, NBC aired an hour-long documentary called *DPT: Vaccine Roulette* that galvanized a nation. For the most part, childhood immunization used to be perceived as a rite of passage and mandatory for school attendance, but the television program portrayed a very different side of the issue.

The show revealed brain-damaged children struggling with daily routines and their frustrated and angry parents lashing out against the vaccine industry and the medical establishment. Many of these parents are famous and powerful individuals, including congressmen and celebrities. The program also included interviews with medical professionals who also seemed to support a link between the DTP vaccine and a host of neurological problems, including convulsions, mental retardation, and behavioral problems.

 Fact

Dissatisfied Parents Together, or DPT, was formed in 1982 by a group of parents who were convinced that vaccines had caused their children to become disabled. This group is now known as the National Vaccine Information Center, and they continue to fight for and promote a vaccine-free society.

Suddenly, parents all over the country started questioning the safety of vaccines. A few parents immediately formed political groups and nonprofit organizations to warn other parents about the danger of immunization. In particular, the focus was on the old DTP vaccine. This vaccine was an easy target because side effects from it were generally more common than those from other vaccines. Swelling and redness at the site of the injection, fever, and pain occurred in close to half of the children receiving the vaccine. In addition, it was well known to the medical community (but not necessarily to most parents) that convulsion, staring spells, and excessive crying were possible complications of the vaccine as well. Though these frightening side effects were less common, the mere fact that they did occur and doctors knew about them left many parents feeling betrayed.

The False Cause Fallacy

Emotions run high on both sides of the vaccine safety debate—the pediatricians who staunchly support vaccination and the parents with disabled children. Both camps routinely downplay the risk of the opponents' arguments and exaggerate the reason for their own thinking. Doctors are often guilty of portraying the worst-case scenario for an infection, even if the particularly serious complication is rare. Parents tend to focus on the devastation of their disabled children, and the purported link between the vaccination and the disability is often just a temporal one.

The cornerstone of the antivaccine argument is that many serious conditions, including autism, sudden infant death syndrome (SIDS), and epilepsy, start manifesting themselves very shortly after these children receive their immunizations. In addition, the number of children diagnosed with autism rose sharply in the 1970s. This time period correlates perfectly to when the MMR combination vaccine was first widely used. Citing these correlations and perfect timing, many parents concluded that vaccines must be responsible for these disabilities.

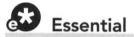 **Essential**

The human mind learns by observation, and one of the most useful types of observation is a temporal relationship between two events. This means that if you see your child throw up after eating mango for the very first time, you are naturally going to conclude that the mango is probably the culprit for the vomiting. This is understandable and logical, and this relationship works most of the time.

At the same time, you can easily relate to the fact that a temporal relationship does not necessarily mean there is a cause-and-effect relationship between two events. In other words, correlation does not imply causation. For example, as ice cream sales increase during the hot summer months, the rate of drowning deaths increases sharply. However, most people would agree that ice cream consumption does not cause drowning. For another example, carbon dioxide levels in the atmosphere increased dramatically in the

1950s, which correlated perfectly to the rapid rise of violent crimes at the same time. But it would be difficult to convince anyone that carbon dioxide caused people to commit violent crimes. A temporal relationship clearly does not imply a causal relationship.

Calculated Risks

The medical community is often guilty of downplaying the risks of vaccination. Doctors usually claim that childhood immunization is completely safe and that there is no reason to worry when your children get immunized. This is not true, and doctors know that this is not true.

Why would your doctor lie to you then? The reason behind the untruth is not malice but a misguided attempt at oversimplification of a very complex problem. The fact is that vaccines are generally safe, but they can cause serious problems in a few individuals receiving them. Why doesn't your doctor tell you about this small risk? Because divulging the answer requires a lengthy explanation that the doctor does not have the time for. Fortunately, you have this book, which will explore all the risks in detail.

Risk Assessment

The fact of the matter is that there are risks in everything you do. When you get up and take a shower in the morning, there is risk in burning yourself with scalding water if you adjust the shower knob incorrectly. There is risk in electrocution when you use a hair dryer to dry your hair near the sink. A car accident could end your life or seriously maim you during your commute. There are countless workplace hazards even if your job does not require you to routinely put yourself in a dangerous situation.

Your children face many of the same hazards. Motor vehicle crashes kill more children than any disease (according to the CDC; see *www.cdc.gov/ncipc/factsheets/childpas.htm*). When you give your daughter Tylenol (acetaminophen) for a fever, there is risk in accidentally overdosing her if she is taking another over-the-counter medication that contains similar ingredients. Even when you give antibiotics to your child for an ear infection, there is the risk of triggering a serious intestinal complication that can lead to death or chronic inflammation.

Even though you are aware of these risks, you commit to these activities anyway because the benefit of these actions outweighs the risks. You are constantly balancing the scale between risk and benefit for everything you do.

The use of seat belts in automobiles is a good way to examine the concept of risk. Seat belts are proven to save lives. The mandatory use of seat belts was introduced in many areas after the dramatic impact of seat belts in reducing mortality in motor vehicle accidents was proven.

🅮 Fact

A study in Sweden showed that no deaths occurred among front-seat passengers wearing seat belts in 28,780 motor vehicle accidents, even at speeds up to 60 miles per hour. Passengers without seat belts were killed at impact speeds as low as 12 miles per hour.

You probably do not need to be convinced of the importance in using seat belts. But are you aware that every time you put on your seat belt in the car you are putting yourself and your children at risk for serious injury by wearing the seat belt?

For example, the use of seat belts has changed the pattern of injuries sustained in motor vehicle accidents. In particular, blunt abdominal trauma has been noted in seat belt wearers. A large Canadian study showed that among seat belt wearers there is an increased risk of intestinal injury resulting directly from the seat belt. The seat belt can cut the small intestine or the spinal cord in half and also cause the spleen to explode during a collision. These complications are obvious life-threatening injuries that require emergency surgical intervention to fix.

Nevertheless, not using the seat belt puts you at even greater risk of serious injuries or death. Naturally, you pick the lesser of two evils and accept the smaller adverse effect of using the seat belt. It's all about balancing the risk and benefit.

The same line of thinking can be applied to vaccines. It is undeniable that vaccines can be dangerous, but the danger of being infected by vaccine-preventable diseases is greater. If there is a way to protect children with risk-free vaccines, the world would no doubt immediately adopt such measure. But a risk-free vaccine, just like a risk-free seat belt, will probably never be invented.

Mercury Preservative

Mercury is indeed a toxic and dangerous substance. When a pregnant mother eats too much mercury while the brain of the unborn child is developing, the baby can suffer permanent brain damage. No amount of mercury in the body is safe. Even a small amount could potentially be harmful.

The Two Faces of Mercury

At the same time, it is important to distinguish between the form of mercury most commonly found in industrial compounds and the mercury used in vaccine preservatives. While both of these chemicals are mercury, they are actually quite different. How can two chemicals containing mercury be so different? It turns out that a little difference in chemistry can make a big difference in how harmful a substance can be.

For example, iron is an essential element for the human body. In order for your body to function properly, you must consume a diet rich in iron. Your body also actively stores iron in case a steady supply of iron is temporarily unavailable from your diet. You have probably heard of anemia resulting from having low level of iron in the body.

However, the iron in your body can only exist safely in some form. Typically the iron is incorporated into other compounds (such as hemoglobin in your blood cells) in order for it to carry out crucial roles in your body's metabolism. At the same time, if the iron gets released from organic compounds in the body and exists alone, it can wreak havoc on the body. Unincorporated iron in the body creates dangerous chemical reactions that can lead to cancer, organ damage, or even death. This essential mineral can be useful in one form and yet be detrimental in another form. A slight difference in chemistry can make the biggest difference in the world when it comes to its biological effect in the human body.

Essential

There are two forms of mercury present in the environment—methyl mercury and ethyl mercury. Most toxicology studies were done on methyl mercury, the form of mercury found in industrial products. Little was known about ethyl mercury, which is present in thimerosal.

Thimerosal in Vaccines

Thimerosal has been a hot topic in vaccine safety for a while, but the debate is quieting down because it is rapidly becoming a moot point in the controversy. This is because of a government mandate in 1997 to remove all traces of mercury preservative from childhood immunizations. By 2001, none of the immunizations given to children under ten contained thimerosal. Nevertheless, a brief discussion is still included in this book because of the abundance of outdated misinformation still circulating in the press and on the Internet.

It is worth noting that the decision to remove the trace amount of mercury from childhood vaccines was not made because a proven link between the mercury preservative and neurological problems. In fact, there have been numerous studies since 2001 that have shown the absence of any association between the mercury-based preservatives in vaccines and autism. The decision to remove the mercury preservative was made because the controversy surrounding the issue was generating panic among parents, and many of them have stopped seeking medical care because of this concern. In order to put everyone's mind at ease, doctors across the country elected to remove all traces of mercury from vaccines.

🔔 Alert

Many Internet resources have not been kept up to date. There are many websites that warn concerned parents about the danger of mercury poisoning. The fact is that there has not been any trace of mercury in any childhood vaccines since 2001.

Ironically, thimerosal was originally added to vaccines to improve vaccine safety. In 1942, eleven children died from a bacteria-contaminated batch of tetanus vaccine. Thimerosal was chosen as the preservative to reduce bacterial contamination because it was deemed safe and effective. The amount of mercury present in teething tablets in the 1960s was more than a hundred times higher than the mercury present in vaccines, so it was determined that the tiny amount of mercury preservative was quite harmless.

Even more interestingly, the pioneer who first brought up the concern of mercury toxicity in vaccines is a pediatrician. Dr. Neal Halsey was the chairman of infectious diseases for the AAP and he has extensive experience working at the CDC on vaccine safety. In 1999, he realized that there might be a potential danger for mercury preservative in vaccines because thimerosal is present in many childhood vaccines. Due to the increase in the number of vaccines children got in the 1990s, the amount of thimerosal injected into children during the first year was several times higher than a decade ago. He also observed that the number of children being diagnosed with speech delay and autism rose sharply during the same period of time. He was concerned, and he started contacting experts in the field to find out whether children were being poisoned during their childhood immunization.

Essential

The fact that a prominent pediatrician stepped forward and loudly provided a dissenting voice when vaccine safety was raised is reassuring that doctors are not usually meek and timid when it comes to protecting their patients' welfare.

At the time Dr. Halsey brought this concern to the attention of the medical community, no one had seriously looked into the question of whether thimerosal was safe or not. It was assumed that it was not toxic because so little of it is present in vaccines. Since the inquiry started, numerous research studies have proven that ethyl mercury is much less toxic than methyl mercury, and the amount that was present in vaccines was harmless.

Fact

It is also important to note that since thimerosal was removed from vaccines, the number of children being diagnosed with autism continued to rise. This rising trend would indicate that whatever is causing autism in children is still in the environment, but thimerosal certainly wasn't the culprit.

However, this is a moot point now, because thimerosal has been removed from all childhood vaccines since 2000. It is important to note that the thimerosal preservative was not removed because it was demonstrated to be harmful, but it was taken out of vaccines because its presence was causing so much anxiety in doctors and parents that it was preventing children from getting vaccinated.

Aluminum Additive

There is growing concern about the safety of aluminum additive in childhood vaccines. Aluminum has been added to vaccines since 1926, and it was originally included in vaccines because scientists ascertained that vaccines containing aluminum work much better than the ones without. Essentially, if aluminum is removed from vaccines today, many of the existing vaccines would not work anymore. Vaccines that include aluminum additive include the hepatitis B vaccine, the DTaP vaccine, the Hib vaccine, and the pneumococcal vaccines.

Exactly how aluminum helps to boost the immune response is not clear. It is hypothesized that the small amount of aluminum causes a minor irritation to the body, which helps alert the immune system to react to the germ-specific components of the vaccine.

It is clearly proven that the aluminum additive in vaccines is responsible for the redness and pain at the injection site for certain vaccines. Even though painful injection is unpleasant, parents are most worried about the long-term problems that may result from aluminum poisoning.

What Is Aluminum?

Aluminum is the most common metal found on this planet. It is ubiquitous. Because it is present in large quantities in the soil, it is absorbed constantly by all living things. Plants and animals all contain traces of this heavy metal. It is also present in breast milk, because mothers get aluminum from the foods and water they consume. The only way to avoid getting aluminum in the body is to stop eating and drinking altogether.

Aluminum is also the main ingredient in many over-the-counter antacids. It is also found in trace amounts in the food you eat every day, because it is present in the soil and is absorbed by plants. In addition, aluminum products are all around you, including many household products, cookware, foil, and construction material. It would be impossible to eliminate your contact with aluminum.

Essential

An exclusively breast-fed baby gets 7 milligrams of aluminum from the breast milk, which is almost twice as much the baby gets from childhood immunization (4.4 milligrams) during the first six months. Formula-fed infants are exposed to even higher amounts of aluminum, up to 117 milligrams, during the first six months of life.

Aluminum Safety

How about the safety profile of aluminum? Just like all heavy metals, aluminum can cause serious problems if present in high levels in the body. You are probably already familiar with the dangerous effects of lead poisoning and mercury toxicity. The good news is that even though all people have aluminum in their bodies, the concentration is very low and does not pose any threat to your health.

Aluminum does not accumulate in the body. Once it is introduced, it is quickly removed from the bloodstream and gets dumped into the urine and out of the body. Because aluminum is excreted through the kidneys, people with reduced kidney functions (that is, those who require dialysis) are most susceptible to aluminum poisoning. Aluminum toxicity rarely occurs in healthy individuals because a tremendous amount of aluminum must be ingested for toxic effects to occur.

When people are exposed to large quantities of aluminum, the effects of aluminum poisoning have been observed. The symptoms include weakened bones, anemia, and brain damage. Dementia has been associated with chronic exposure to aluminum, with the victim manifesting symptoms similar to Alzheimer's disease. However, this only occurs when the level of aluminum in the body rises to thousands of times that of an average individual.

Despite decades of use in vaccines, the trace amount of aluminum introduced into the body has never caused any identifiable harmful effect. The bottom line is that the extremely small amount of aluminum added to vaccines does not pose any health risk for children and adults. Relative to our constant exposure to aluminum from other sources, the amount of aluminum in vaccines is miniscule.

 Fact

> In 2000, the World Health Organization examined the level of aluminum in childhood immunization. They found no evidence of toxicity because the concentration of aluminum is extremely low in vaccines.

The important thing to remember is that anything can be toxic to the human body if present in large enough quantities. Even drinking excessive water can cause seizure and death. With the abundance of information, you must interpret the data with the proper perspective. Just because iron can be extremely toxic to the body doesn't mean you should stop eating food rich in iron. Your body needs a small amount of iron to function properly. Without it, you will suffer from severe anemia or death. While a small amount of iron is beneficial to the body, a high level of iron is extremely toxic and can lead to liver failure, heart failure, and death. In fact, iron poisoning is the leading cause of poisoning deaths in children. But just because iron is toxic in high concentration doesn't mean it is dangerous in small quantities. The same is true for aluminum.

How to Protect Your Child

It is probably safe to assume that most doctors did not become doctors so that they could intentionally harm and kill children. You have to trust that doctors would not endorse and administer vaccines to children if they believe vaccination is inherently detrimental to your child's health. What would doctors gain by intentionally making your child sick? Why would doctors allow their own children to be vaccinated if they believe the procedure is inherently harmful?

Finding a Trusted Source

When it comes down to it, your doctor is the only source of information you can trust. That being said, if you do not feel comfortable with your doctor or do not trust her 100 percent, it is time to look for a new doctor.

 Alert

Anyone can post information on the Internet. A website costs six dollars a month to maintain and about two days to set up. Most websites have a hidden agenda. Do not trust information on the Internet, because anything you read could be completely made up.

Each vaccine has its unique risk and benefit. Instead of relying on information from the Internet, talk to a doctor you can trust. A good doctor should spend the time necessary to explain all of your concerns about each vaccine and answer all of your questions. If your doctor will not or cannot do that, switch to another provider. Your child's life is at stake here, and you need the most knowledgeable and compassionate advocate on your side. Arming yourself with the most reliable information and making an informed decision based on that information is the best gift you can give to your child.

Reconciliation and Cooperation

People involved in the fray of vaccine controversy often forget that the two sides of the vaccine battle really should be working together instead of fighting each other. What is most difficult to achieve for both sides is for each to listen dispassionately to the other side and temporarily put one's own agenda aside. After all, it is important to remember that the two sides of the camp are really after one common goal—the well-being of children.

Doctors need to listen to the parents without being condescending or impatient. In addition, they must not take it personally when parents decline their recommended vaccine schedule. Medical professionals must understand that these parents are not disparaging them but are only doing what they believe is best for the most important people in their lives. Many physicians today dismiss patients from their practice if the parents decline vaccination for their children, but the practice of "firing" parents from practices must stop. These are not parents who neglect or abuse their children, and their wish to look after the best interest for their children must be encouraged and supported.

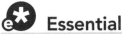 **Essential**

Very few doctors would ever want to intentionally harm their patients. Doctors get angry when parents decline their recommendation because they perceive that the parents must not trust their judgment or ethical standard.

On the other hand, well-intentioned parents must remember that pediatricians are not merely pawns of the pharmaceutical industry. There is nothing for doctors to gain by knowingly recommending something that is harmful to children. The lifelong mission for all pediatricians is to protect the welfare of children and be their most steadfast advocate. If you have second thoughts about trusting your pediatrician, you should find another doctor that you can completely trust.

Finally, doctors are trained to question the established way of doing things. Medical advances depend on medical personnel challenging the authority and considering better alternatives. If it weren't for the inquisitive minds of many brilliant doctors, modern medicine would be no different from the way medicine was practiced hundreds of years ago. The fact that the immunization schedule has been changed almost yearly testifies to this sentiment.

In the best of all possible worlds, galvanized parents and compassionate physicians would work together to find better ways to prevent sickness and suffering in children. Whether this should be done by the current immunization standard or other alternatives should be continuously investigated as the epidemics of infection changes. An open mind with a relentless drive is the only path to victory in the constant battle between humanity and germs.

CHAPTER 5

Vaccines and Autism

One of the greatest controversies surrounding vaccines is whether immunization can trigger autism in children. This is a highly emotional topic because autism is such a devastating condition. Parents of autistic children understandably feel strongly about this topic, and they often find themselves at odds with the established medical practice. What makes it even more difficult is that most doctors do not lend a sympathetic ear to listen to their perspective. This chapter will dissect the topic and the controversy without getting mired in emotional arguments.

What Is Autism?

Autism is a neurological condition that interferes with a person's ability to communicate and relate to other people. It is not a single disease but rather a description for a group of disorders that affect people in similar ways. This group of conditions is often referred to as autism spectrum disorders (ASD). Some autistic people are better at using language than others, while others may not speak a single word throughout their entire lives.

A milder form of autism is called Asperger's syndrome. For people with Asperger's syndrome, their linguistic skills remain largely intact, yet they still have a hard time reading social cues and understanding subtle humor, such as irony or cynicism.

People with Asperger's syndrome tend to interpret situations literally, and they like to stick to routines.

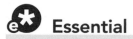 Fact

In addition to Asperger's syndrome, the autism spectrum disorders also include conditions such as Rett syndrome, pervasive developmental disorder, and childhood disintegrative disorder. It is beyond the scope of this book to explain in detail each of these conditions.

There is hardly anything more profoundly devastating than having an autistic child, even though it can be rewarding at times to see your child making gradual progress. After going through the normal stages of grief—denial, anger, bargaining, depression, and finally acceptance—each parent eventually comes to terms with autism and accepts the daily challenges and deals with them one day at a time.

Essential

In the film *Rain Man*, Dustin Hoffman portrayed a fictional autistic man with a photographic memory and astounding artistic abilities. In real life, however, most autistic individuals do not possess superhuman talents, and the vast majority need additional help to carry out the activities of daily living.

An autistic child requires constant supervision, no matter the age. There is never a day off from autism, and the accumulation of stress adds to the burden. If you ever thought that raising a typical toddler is a challenge, you have no idea what dealing with an autistic child is like. Every parent loves his autistic child, but sometimes the behaviors associated with this disease can frustrate even the most patient person.

Autism robs a child of the ability to relate and empathize. It is very difficult for autistic children to reach out and connect with others. This is most apparent when autism interferes with linguistic skills, but it affects children on many levels. Autistic children cannot easily relate to the feelings of others, and they find it very difficult to make their needs known to others.

A Day with Autism

To give parents of nonautistic children some understanding of what it is like to spend a day with a child with autism, here is an account of a typical day in a household with two parents and their autistic son. Even though this is not a real household, the anecdotes are based on real life events.

 Fact

Boys are more likely to be diagnosed with ASD than girls. Why this is the case is not entirely clear to doctors and scientists.

Jake is six years old. He woke up at 4:30 A.M. the usual way, screaming at the top of his lungs in his room. His parents, Jeremy and Linda, are used to this by now, so they no longer rush into the room fearing the worst.

It took Jeremy forty-five minutes to get Jake out of his pajamas and into his daytime clothes, all the while Jake screamed and kicked, protesting this mundane daily routine. In the meantime, Linda was getting Jake's breakfast ready, breaking open a capsule and sprinkling the powder in Jake's oatmeal so he could get his morning medication as part of his breakfast. She also had to get the placemat and the chair placed just so. Jake would have a meltdown if things are not exactly positioned the way they always are.

Breakfast was not so bad on this particular day. Jake actually ate most of his oatmeal (along with his medication that allows him to focus better in school) and got into the car seat willingly. It was already 6:45 A.M. and Jeremy dropped Jake off at school.

By 11:30 A.M., Linda got a call from school. Jake's teacher said that Jake had spat at other children and he would not stop doing so. Linda drove to the school and picked him up. Since Jake does not talk at all, Linda spent half an hour in vain asking him to stop. Jake spat on his mother's face a few times before he quit the behavior.

Linda took Jake home anyway, because he has an appointment with his pediatric developmentalist in the afternoon. The appointment was uneventful, except that Jake almost hit another child in the waiting room before they were called into the exam room. Fortunately, the spitting did not resume.

On the way back to their car, Jake broke free from his mother and dashed around in the parking lot. Linda chased after him, but Jake was nearly hit by a car backing out of the lot. It was a good thing that the driver was alert and stepped on the brake just in time to avoid running Jake over.

Back home, Linda spent the rest of the afternoon reinforcing the skills that were introduced today earlier at the doctor's office. It was slow, and Jake did not seem to make any progress.

Linda does not work. Her life is consumed by Jake's behavior, doctor appointments, home therapy, and the constant supervision. She has not worked since Jake was diagnosed with autism at the age of twenty-six months. She gave up her lucrative career as a public relations officer at a large software firm to devote all of her time and energy to taking care of Jake.

To be fair, there are occasional small rewards for Linda and Jeremy. Every now and then, Jake surprises them by spontaneously showing some gesture of appreciation. In sporadic spurts, Jake manages to learn new skills that make going through the daily grind a bit easier. Linda and Jeremy cling to these golden moments tenaciously.

The last four years have taken a toll on both Linda and Jeremy, and they are going to marriage counseling twice a month to keep the relationship from falling apart. Jeremy filed for divorce last year, but they did not go through with it. They no longer feel like the loving couple they used to be. They are emotionally drained by Jake's constant needs, and they occasionally vent their frustration and stress by lashing out at one another.

What happened to their hopes and dreams of raising their son and watching him go to college? What is going to happen to Jake when he becomes an adult? What are the odds that they will ever be grandparents?

How Autism Is Diagnosed

Scientists and doctors are getting better and better at diagnosing autism. One reason for the improvement in diagnosis is that autism is far more common today than in the past. Back in the 1940s, when autism was first recognized as a psychiatric disorder, autism was thought to be a very rare condition, affecting less than 1 in 10,000 children. Over the years, especially during the early 1990s, the number of reported cases of autism soared. Initially, most clinicians believed that this increase was due to increased awareness of the condition and that doctors were finally diagnosing autism correctly in children. In the past, most of these children might have been labeled as mentally retarded. However, most experts today believe that the actual number of children with autism is on the rise, and better diagnosis does not fully explain the recent rising tide of autism around the world.

Autism can most often be diagnosed by the time the child is three years of age, but some highly trained experts can start identifying autistic traits in children at six months of age. The diagnosis of autism is usually confirmed by a child psychiatrist or other specially trained mental health experts that have experience taking care of autistic children. However, the first sign of autism is most often noticed by the parents. More often than not, parents bring their children to the doctor, claiming that something is just not quite right about their child. What tips the parents off could be the way that their child plays with his toys or that he does not seem to be interested in other children. Delayed speech is a major warning sign.

🅔❗ Alert

Today, about 1 in 150 children in the United States is diagnosed with an autism spectrum disorder. This statistic makes autism one of the most common chronic conditions in childhood.

At first, some doctors may brush off these parental concerns and reassure the parents that the child will just grow out of this phase and eventually catch up to his peers. While this wait-and-see approach may work for some children, it only delays crucial intensive therapy autistic children need to modify and improve their behavior. If you suspect that your child may be autistic, do not hesitate to bring this to your doctor's attention. A simple screening test could either give you peace of mind or provide your child the advantage of an early head start on treatment.

There are many standardized screening tests doctors use to diagnose autism. A popular one is called M-CHAT, which stands for the Modified Checklist for Autism in Toddlers. This checklist asks the parents a string of simple questions about their child's behavior. This screening tool is designed for toddler ages sixteen to thirty months. The checklist is provided here:

Please fill out the following about how your child usually is. Please try to answer every question. If the behavior is rare (e.g. you've seen it once or twice), please answer as if the child does not do it.

1. Does your child enjoy being swung, bounced on your knee, etc.?
2. Does your child take an interest in other children?
3. Does your child like climbing on things, such as up stairs?
4. Does your child enjoy playing peek-a-boo/hide-and-seek?
5. Does your child ever pretend, for example, to talk on the phone or take care of a doll or pretend other things?
6. Does your child ever use his/her index finger to point, to ask for something?
7. Does your child ever use his/her index finger to point, to indicate interest in something?
8. Can your child play properly with small toys (e.g. cars or blocks) without just mouthing, fiddling, or dropping them?
9. Does your child ever bring objects over to you (parent) to show you something?
10. Does your child look you in the eye for more than a second or two?
11. Does your child ever seem oversensitive to noise? (e.g. plugging ears)
12. Does your child smile in response to your face or your smile?
13. Does your child imitate you? (e.g. you make a face—will your child imitate it?)
14. Does your child respond to his/her name when you call?
15. If you point at a toy across the room, does your child look at it?
16. Does your child walk?
17. Does your child look at things you are looking at?
18. Does your child make unusual finger movements near his/her face?
19. Does your child try to attract your attention to his/her own activity?

20. Have you ever wondered if your child is deaf?
21. Does your child understand what people say?
22. Does your child sometimes stare at nothing or wander with no purpose?
23. Does your child look at your face to check your reaction when faced with something unfamiliar?

© 1999 Diana Robins, Deborah Fein, & Marianne Barton

An answer is considered critical if you responded "Yes" to questions 11, 18, 20, and 22 and "No" to all the other questions. If you have more than three critical answers to any of the questions or more than two critical answers to questions 2, 7, 9, 13, 14, and 15, the risk is higher that your child may be diagnosed with ASD.

🔔 Alert

It is very important to keep in mind that the M-CHAT is only a screening tool, which means if your child scored a high risk for ASD, it does not mean that she has autism. There are many children who get a high score using the M-CHAT questionnaire and are later found by an expert not to have ASD.

If the results from the M-CHAT indicate your child is at high risk for being diagnosed with ASD, talk to your doctor immediately. Remember that the M-CHAT is only a screening tool, so having a high-risk score does not necessarily mean that your child has autism. Nevertheless, consultation with an expert is appropriate if the scoring puts your child in a high-risk area.

What Causes Autism?

The cause of autism is the source of many controversies, mainly because it is largely unknown at this time. Historically, when doctors were just starting to understand autism, many physicians believed that autism was the result of poor parenting techniques. Ironically, one of the pioneers of autism, Dr. Leo Kanner at Johns Hopkins University, first described the "refrigerator mother" theory as the cause of autism. He concluded that autistic children seem detached to other people because their mothers failed to show warmth during their upbringing. What he observed was that the parents of autistic children did not have a lot of interaction with their children, and he deduced the lack of interaction could contribute to the lack of social skills in these children. What he did not take into consideration is the fact that these parents demonstrated little interaction with their children only because these children regularly turned away their affection. After a long period of time, these parents learned to keep their distance and avoid close personal interaction with the children.

 Fact

If autism is purely genetic, there would not be an increase in the number of diagnoses made. An epidemic is triggered by some external factor. A purely genetic condition simply cannot have a sudden global epidemic of autism.

Fortunately, we now know that parents are not to blame for causing their children to be autistic. Nevertheless, there is strong evidence that autism is partly caused by genetic factors. Several facts led to this conclusion. Siblings of autistic children are much more likely to be diagnosed with autism, and autistic traits tend to run in families. Recently several genes have been identified that predispose children to have autistic tendencies.

Even though the burden of poor parenting has been lifted from parents, a genetic cause still makes many parents feel somewhat responsible for their children's plight. The guilt is not intentional, but somehow they feel blamed because the seed of autism could have come from themselves.

It is also obvious that genetics does not explain the whole story. If autism is purely inherited, you would expect all autistic children to have autistic parents, or at least autistic relatives. This is definitely not the case. So on top of having a genetic predisposition, there is something else that seems to trigger the onset of autism. It is this "something else" that is at the heart of the controversy.

Unfortunately, no one knows what the triggers are for autism. In all likelihood, there are numerous triggers that can possibly cause autism. Autism is probably the end result of a combination of genetic factors and environmental triggers. Some have hypothesized that a defective immune system plays a role in triggering autism, while others blamed environmental pollutants. Some even lay the blame on vitamin deficiency. Many parents believe that childhood vaccination plays a role in triggering autism in some children.

The MMR Vaccine and Autism

The current concern about the MMR vaccine and its association with autism is based on three things. The first was an observation that the number of children diagnosed with autism increased dramatically right around the same time the MMR combination vaccine was introduced in the United States and Great Britain. The second was based on a study by Dr. Andrew Wakefield in 1998 published in the respected scientific journal *Lancet*. The third is based on the fact that children with autism were first diagnosed with the condition right after they received the MMR vaccine.

To look at the first link, it is obvious that the number of children diagnosed with autism increased dramatically around the same time the MMR vaccine was given to many children. The MMR combination vaccine first became available in 1971. Back in the 1970s, 1 in 10,000 children was diagnosed with autism. Currently, it is estimated that 1 in 150 children is expected to have the diagnosis. The timing of the two events could not have correlated better. Many parents looked at this perfect timing and concluded that the MMR vaccine must be responsible for triggering the current global epidemic of autism in developed countries.

However, there are some problems with this association because the way autism was diagnosed changed after the MMR vaccine was introduced, leading to more children being diagnosed as autistic. Prior to the early 1990s, autism had a more narrow definition. The definition of autism changed twice between 1987 and 1994 in the *Diagnostic and Statistical Manual of Mental Disorders* (DSM). The DSM-III-R and DSM-IV (third edition, revised, and fourth edition, respectively) gave a much more precise definition of autism, thereby allowing clinicians to make a more accurate diagnosis of autism instead of classifying some of these children as mentally retarded as was done in the past. Consequently, more autistic children are being diagnosed correctly today than ever before.

In addition, autism was not a well-known condition prior to the 1980s. Most doctors were not familiar with this condition and therefore could not correctly identify children with autism before that time. Another event that resulted from this increased public awareness was the increasing availability of public services, both in school and in the community, for these children. Consequently, more children are getting diagnosed earlier and correctly so they can qualify for these special assistant programs. Even though the rise of autism occurred around the same time as the MMR vaccine was first introduced to the public, it is unclear that one event led to the other.

The second link between the MMR vaccine and autism was established by the famous study done by Dr. Wakefield published in *Lancet*. Dr. Wakefield is a Canadian surgeon who studied twelve children in 1998 who purportedly became developmentally delayed after receiving the MMR vaccine. His hypothesis is that the

MMR vaccine can trigger inflammation in the intestine, and this inflammation can subsequently allow harmful proteins to enter the bloodstream and the brain. He theorized that autism is the effect of these harmful proteins on the brain. He was the original doctor who proposed that the MMR vaccine should be separated into individual vaccines to prevent intestinal inflammation, even though there is no evidence that separating the vaccines makes any difference to the immune system.

⊕ Alert

Dr. Andrew Wakefield is currently under legal indictment by the British General Medical Council for professional misconduct. Prior to making the statement that endorses separating the MMR vaccine into individual vaccines, he filed a patent for an individualized measles vaccine, which means he could reap financial gains from widespread use of this single measles vaccine.

To prove his theory, in 2002 he took biopsies from a group of autistic children's intestines and demonstrated the presence of measles virus in the intestinal cells. He found that most autistic children (75 out of 91) have measles virus in the intestinal tissue and that most nonautistic children (65 out of 70) do not have the measles virus in their intestines. This result certainly sounds convincing that the measles virus could somehow be related to autism.

The question is whether the measles virus found in these autistic children's intestines came from the vaccines or from natural measles infection. At the time of the study, measles outbreaks still occurred fairly frequently in Britain, where the study took place. Even though Dr. Wakefield could determine whether the measles virus found in autistic children's intestines was the weakened version from the vaccine or the regular kind from natural infection, he chose not to do so. In addition, recent investigation revealed that Dr. Wakefield had fabricated experimental data in order to support his hypothesis. Most of the coauthors of Dr. Wakefield's published research have since withdrawn their names and support from the report in *Lancet.*

 Fact

Ten of the twelve authors of Dr. Wakefield's research later retracted their original conclusion that the MMR vaccine could be implicated in causing autism. The retraction states that no causal link was established between the MMR vaccine and autism.

On the other hand, Japanese scientists (led by Dr. Hideo Honda) had demonstrated in 2005 that children continued to develop autism even when the MMR vaccine was no longer given to an entire group of children. Due to a concern about a possible side effect of the mumps vaccine, the MMR vaccine was no longer recommend for children in the city of Yokohama (population 300,000) from 1988 to 1996. Starting in 1993, not a single shot of the MMR vaccine was given in the entire city. Despite the fact that the MMR vaccination had completely stopped, the number of autistic children continued to rise in the city. In fact, the number of new diagnoses since 1993 nearly doubled compared to the time period before the MMR vaccine was stopped. This clearly demonstrates that children continue to become autistic at an alarming rate even if they have never received the MMR vaccine.

Finally, there is an obvious reason why autism is almost always diagnosed after the MMR vaccine is administered. In order to diagnose autism, speech and social interaction with other children are key diagnostic criteria. Even normal, nonautistic children typically do not have fluent speech before they turn one. In addition, social interactions of infants are typically limited. Autistic children only stand out when the language skills of their nonautistic peers really start to take off. This developmental milestone occurs right around the time when the first MMR vaccine is given.

One convincing fact that makes this temporal relationship unlikely to be a causal one is that autism can sometimes be diagnosed by experienced experts when these children are only six months old. This is far before these children receive their first MMR vaccine. By the time these children who are identified early receive their first MMR shot, they are already autistic. The timing explanation does not work if children were autistic without ever receiving the MMR vaccine.

To this day, scientists do not know exactly which factors can trigger autism. It is clear that it is a strongly genetic condition. It is also clear that autism could be diagnosed before the age of one and before receiving the first MMR vaccine. Finally, even when one entire community stopped administering the MMR vaccine, many children continued to become autistic. These observations make it hard to conclude that the MMR vaccine is solely responsible for the current autism epidemic around the world.

Thimerosal and Autism

The link between thimerosal and autism will soon become a historical footnote. Thimerosal is a mercury-based preservative that was once used in some childhood vaccines prior to 2001. Due to the fear of potential problems resulting from this preservative, many parents declined vaccination for their children. Doctors were concerned that infectious outbreaks may start to occur in urban areas when too few people are vaccinated, so to encourage vaccination and reassure parents, thimerosal was removed from all childhood vaccines in 2001. For more discussion on the history and safety of thimerosal, please refer to Chapter 4 on vaccine safety.

Since the removal of the thimerosal preservative from vaccines, the number of children diagnosed with autism continues to rise sharply. If thimerosal were a trigger for autism, far fewer children would have been diagnosed with autism since 2000, when the preservative was removed. Unfortunately, this is not what happened.

Since 2001, more and more children are diagnosed as autistic than ever before.

It would be wonderful if thimerosal were the culprit for the autism epidemic—removing it from vaccines would have stopped this childhood plague of the modern world. But autism has proven to be more complex than that. Getting rid of thimerosal has done nothing to halt the global autism epidemic.

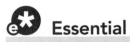 **Essential**

It is important to understand that thimerosal was removed from childhood vaccines not because it has caused problems but because of the concern associated with it scaring parents and many parents deciding not to vaccinate their children at all. The reduced immunization had already spurred whooping cough and measles outbreaks around the world.

Autism Treatment

Since this book is not a book on autism, this section can only provide limited information on the treatment options for autistic children. Autism is a permanent neurological condition that affects language and behavior. It would be hard to say that there is a "cure" for autism. While intense speech therapy and behavioral intervention can drastically improve the behavior and communication skills of an autistic child, children with autism will probably never be as independent as children without autism. Many adults with high-functioning autism live independently, have rewarding careers, and even have families. At the same time, these high-functioning autistic adults still have characteristics that set them apart from their nonautistic peers. They tend to be more aloof, and they are frequently most comfortable when they are alone. There is certain degree of awkwardness in social settings.

⊛ Essential

A popular approach to behavioral modification for autistic children is a method called *applied behavior analysis*. This general strategy can be utilized in other arenas such as training athletes, environmental conservation, and parenting.

If you are concerned your child may have some autistic traits, the first thing to do is to talk to your pediatrician. If the doctor shares your concern, your child should be referred to a child behavioral expert for further evaluation. The key to successful intervention in helping your child reach his potential is an early start on the treatment. Intensive speech therapy and behavioral modification programs are necessary to help your child gain valuable skills, and the earlier these programs are instituted, the better your child will do in the future.

CHAPTER 6

Current Immunization Schedule

The immunization schedule constantly changes from year to year. It is updated annually (and sometimes more frequent than that) to adapt to the introduction of new vaccines and the elimination of old ones. It is a daunting task to stay on top of all the new changes, even for medical professionals. You may find this chapter to be the most technical part of the book, and don't be discouraged if you do not remember everything that is covered in this chapter. Keep this book as a reference whenever you need a reminder for a specific vaccine or situation.

Infancy

Your infant child is scheduled to receive more vaccines during the first twelve months than any other time in her life. This busy schedule is necessary because the first twelve months is a very special time in your child's life. Her immune system is not quite mature, yet there is an increasing number of germs waiting to breach her immune system when she becomes more mobile and explores the world. The first twelve months of your baby's life is also the most vulnerable time of her life. She needs all the help she can get when it comes to fending off germs.

Due to the recent invention of many new vaccines, the number of shots steadily increased in the past twenty years. New vaccines such as the hepatitis A vaccine, the pneumococcal conjugate vaccine, and the rotavirus vaccine were all introduced for infants in the past twenty years.

There may be minor variations in vaccination schedule between various medical offices. Since there is a window of time when the baby is recommended to receive many of the vaccines, each medical practice may tailor the immunization schedule to fit into the flow of the practice and appointment availability. Consult your doctor for the specific schedule that the medical practice is following.

Birth

The first vaccine your baby receives is usually the hepatitis B vaccine. This vaccine is now routinely given to newborn babies in the hospital within the first two days after birth. The hepatitis B vaccine is given so early in the life because it can protect babies from hepatitis B if their mothers are carriers for the hepatitis B virus. If a newborn baby gets hepatitis B, she almost always becomes afflicted with the most serious complications of the hepatitis B infection, which include liver failure and liver cancer.

 Fact

The hepatitis B vaccine is also unique in that it is the only vaccine that is approved to be given at birth. The minimum age for most other vaccines is six weeks of age.

If your baby did not receive the hepatitis B vaccine in the hospital after birth, he can still get the vaccine at the two-month visit. If your doctor administers combination vaccines that include the hepatitis B vaccine, it is okay to get a total of four doses of the hepatitis B vaccine.

Two Months

When your baby is two months old, she is due for her next set of shots. These usually include the second hepatitis B vaccine, the combination DTaP vaccine, the Hib vaccine, the pneumococcal conjugate vaccine, the polio vaccine, and the rotavirus vaccine. Many of these vaccines are available in combination injections, so your child might not receive all six vaccines individually.

Even though these vaccines are usually given at the two-month well baby visit, they can be given as early as six weeks after birth. If your baby was born prematurely, she still follows the same schedule as a full-term baby. The timing of the vaccine starts at birth no matter what gestational age your baby was born.

Essential

A common combination vaccine is called Pediarix. This vaccine combines the hepatitis B vaccine, the DTaP vaccine, and the polio vaccine all into one injectable form. Another combination vaccine, called Tri-HIBit, combines the Hib vaccine with the DTaP vaccine. The COMVAX vaccine combines the Hib vaccine with the hepatitis B vaccine.

The rotavirus vaccine does not come in an injectable form. It comes in a liquid form administered through the mouth. Your baby drinks this vaccine, so thankfully there is no pain involved in the process. The schedule for the rotavirus vaccine is also a little tricky. If your baby missed the rotavirus vaccine at two months of age, she cannot get any rotavirus vaccine after twelve weeks of age. This restriction exists because scientists do not have safety information for the vaccine outside of this age range. So if your child did not get the first rotavirus vaccine within this window of opportunity (six to twelve weeks), she can no longer get this vaccine for the rest of her life.

To summarize, at the two-month visit, your baby could get as many as five shots plus an oral vaccine, or as few as three shots plus the oral vaccine. It is possible that in the future more of these vaccines will be further combined into even fewer shots so each visit is easier on your baby and on you.

Four Months

These exact same vaccines are usually administered at the four-month visit. If your baby has had no reaction to these vaccines after the first round, chances are that she is going to be fine again the second time.

The minimum time interval between the first set of shots and the next one is four weeks for babies less than a year old. After the age of one, the second Hib and pneumococcal conjugate vaccines can be given eight weeks after the first dose.

Six Months

Typically, the routine vaccination given at six months of age is the same as the previous two sets at the two- and four-month visit. The vaccines include the DTaP vaccine, the IPV (killed polio) vaccine, the hepatitis B vaccine, the Hib vaccine, the pneumococcal vaccine, and the rotavirus oral vaccine.

 Fact

Since some vaccines can be given at any time within a window of time, there may be some variations in the vaccination schedule among various medical practices. Consult your doctor and ask for a copy of the immunization schedule used at that particular medical office.

In some medical practices where the PRP-OMP Hib vaccine is used rather than the PRP-T Hib variety (please refer to Chapter 10 for details about the different varieties of the Hib conjugate vaccine), the Hib vaccine may be omitted at the six-month visit. In addition, some doctors may elect to postpone the third hepatitis B and polio vaccine until the nine-month visit.

Beside these routine shots, your baby is finally old enough to get the flu shot at six months of age. The flu vaccine is not available throughout the year, so consult your pediatrician for the best time to get your baby the flu shot.

Nine Months

If your child has already gotten the hepatitis B and the polio vaccine during the six-month visit, he would not need to get any shots at the nine-month well baby visit. However, if your child is behind on shots, the nine-month visit provides a good opportunity to catch up on the vaccinations.

There are a handful of vaccines due at the one-year checkup. These vaccines cannot be administered prior to one year of age because they may not work very well if given too early.

Twelve Months

The one-year visit is a tough one for your child (and possibly for you). There are many vaccines scheduled at this visit, and your child may get as many as six vaccines at one time.

The vaccines scheduled at this visit include the DTaP vaccine (fourth dose), the pneumococcal conjugate vaccine (fourth dose), the Hib vaccine (either the third or fourth dose, depending on the type of Hib vaccines given previously), the MMR vaccine (first dose), the chickenpox vaccine (first dose), and the hepatitis A vaccine (first dose).

Your child may not get all six vaccines at this visit because there are some variations in the immunization schedule from one medical practice to the next. The fourth DTaP vaccine must be administered at least six months after the third dose, so some doctors wait until the fifteen- or eighteen-month visit to give the fourth DTaP vaccine. The first hepatitis A vaccine can be given any time between age one and two, so many practices postpone this vaccine until the eighteen-month or two-year appointment.

Due to a national shortage of the Hib vaccine, the current recommendation is to omit the final dose of the Hib vaccine if your child has gotten at least two doses of the PRP-OMP Hib vaccine or at least three doses of the PRP-T Hib vaccine. This is to conserve the existing Hib vaccine that is in short supply for the younger babies who need more protection than the older children.

🅴❗ Alert

When you schedule the appointment for the one-year checkup, make sure you pick a date that is after your child's first birthday. There are some vaccines due at twelve months that cannot be given prior to the first birthday.

Eighteen to Twenty-Four Months

During these visits, the vaccines your child gets may vary quite a bit from one medical office to the other. Depending on what were given at the twelve-month appointment, your child may get anywhere from one to five shots.

If your child has not received the DTaP vaccine or the hepatitis A vaccine at the twelve-month visit, this is the time to get these shots. In addition, if your child is behind on certain vaccines, this is the opportunity to get him caught up. In some practices, the third hepatitis B vaccine is not given until these visits.

Childhood

After the flurry of shots during the first two years of your child's life, he finally gets a break. Usually there is no routine scheduled immunization between the ages of two and four. However, if your child goes to daycare, the daycare may require your child to get tested for tuberculosis through a skin test. This is also called the PPD skin test (PPD stands for purified protein derivative), the tuberculin test, or the Mantoux test (named after the French physician who helped invent this test). This test is not technically a vaccine but a screening test to see who may have been exposed to tuberculosis. This book will not discuss the TB test because it is beyond the topic of vaccine. Talk to your doctor for more information about this test.

Four to Six Years

When your child is ready to enter preschool, the school usually requires a form to be filled out. This form includes a copy of your child's immunization record or a statement that you have declined immunization because it is against your religious or ethical principles.

The four-year vaccination includes the second MMR vaccine, the second chickenpox vaccine, the fifth dose of the DTaP vaccine, and the fourth IPV (killed polio) vaccine. If your child has not gotten the hepatitis A vaccine, this is the time to get that, too.

 Essential

Even though the second MMR vaccine is usually scheduled at the four- to six-year visit, it can be given as early as four weeks after the initial MMR vaccine. If your child has already received two doses of the MMR vaccine (assuming the first dose is given after the first birthday), a third dose would be unnecessary.

Adolescent Years

Many adolescents are not getting the vaccines they need because they are busy with school, and there is no frequent, regularly scheduled visit to the doctor's around this time. Unless they are sick and come to the doctor's office often, they can slip through the cracks and get behind on their immunization needs.

The most common missed vaccine for adolescents is the tetanus booster. The booster given to adolescents is different from the

DTaP vaccine designed for younger children. For children older than eleven, the Tdap booster vaccine is recommended instead. The difference between the childhood DTaP vaccine and the adolescent Tdap vaccine is that the Tdap vaccine contains smaller amounts of the diphtheria and pertussis components.

The capitalization scheme for the DTaP vaccine and the Tdap vaccine actually confers some meaning. The capitalized letter in the name means the vaccine contains a full dose of that particular component. The small letter in the name means that the vaccine contains only a partial dose of a component.

For example, the DTaP means this vaccine has the full dose for the diphtheria, tetanus, and pertussis component. The small a stands for acellular, indicating that this vaccine does not have whole pertussis germ in the vaccine. The Tdap vaccine only contains the full dose of the tetanus vaccine. The letters d and p are not capitalized because the Tdap vaccine contains only partial doses for these two components. The older Td booster had a full dose of the tetanus component but only a partial diphtheria component. The Td booster did not have any pertussis component in the vaccine.

In addition to the Tdap booster, adolescents may have fallen behind on their hepatitis A vaccine and chickenpox booster. The hepatitis A vaccine was not universally recommended when some adolescents were still in their childhood, so they may have never gotten this vaccine. Only one dose of the chickenpox vaccine was given prior to 2006, but the new recommendation suggests two doses for everyone. Therefore, many teens may have only received one dose.

Starting in 2005, a new vaccine for adolescents that prevents meningitis became available. A single dose of the meningococcal vaccine (trade name Menactra) is recommended for all children age eleven to eighteen. Please refer to Chapter 16 for a detailed discussion about this new vaccine.

Finally, the HPV (human papilloma virus) vaccine was introduced in 2006. This vaccine is recommended only for girls between age eleven and twenty-six. Please consult Chapter 17 of this book for a comprehensive description for the HPV vaccine.

Adulthood

Parents usually think of vaccines as something their children get, but adults need to be vaccinated, too. Shots are not just for kids. Chances are that you are behind on your shots if you have not seen your doctor in the past five years.

Young Adults

Just like adolescents, adults need the Tdap booster every ten years for the rest of their life. Since adults are the most common source for whooping cough, staying on top of your immunization may protect your children and grandchildren.

In addition, the HPV vaccine is also recommended for adults up to age twenty-six. After the upper age limit, you can still benefit from the HPV vaccine, but the benefit may be smaller. Talk to your doctor if you are not sure whether you should get the HPV vaccine.

Healthy adults are advised to get the annual flu vaccine. This is especially important if you have chronic problems with your lungs, heart, liver, or kidneys. Older adults over the age of fifty are also recommended for the annual flu vaccine. If you work around young children or people with weakened immune system, you should protect these vulnerable individuals around you by getting the flu shot yourself.

Older Adults

A new vaccine against shingles was especially designed for older adults. It became available in 2006. Shingles is a recurrence of a past chickenpox infection. It occurs when the chickenpox virus that was dormant in the body becomes active again, causing painful blisters to form in one area of the skin. Even though shingles can occur at any age, it is most common for people over the age of fifty.

Even though the shingles vaccine may be beneficial for people younger than sixty, this vaccine has not been tested in the age group younger than sixty. The safety of this vaccine is unknown for younger individuals, therefore this vaccine is not indicated for anyone below the age of sixty.

The new shingles vaccine is similar to the chickenpox vaccine for children, but it is devised differently to protect adults who may already have had the chickenpox infection. It is recommended for anyone over the age of sixty, and only a single dose of the vaccine is needed.

Essential

The shingles vaccine can prevent shingles, but it is useless once shingles occurs. There are other treatments available to alleviate the painful rash of shingles. Consult your doctor for the best therapeutic option for you if you develop shingles.

The pneumococcal polysaccharide vaccine is recommended for individuals older than sixty-five. This vaccine differs from the pneumococcal conjugate vaccine for babies in that it contains components against twenty-three types of the pneumococci bacteria (versus the seven types in the conjugate vaccine). The pneumococcal polysaccharide vaccine is also different from the pneumococcal conjugate vaccine because it does not work well for children younger than age two. The polysaccharide vaccine is also recommended for children older than two if they have a weakened immune system, including sickle cell anemia; people with chronic lung, heart, liver, or kidney diseases; diabetics; alcoholics; people with cancer or AIDS; organ transplant recipients; people without a spleen; and people whose spinal fluid is leaking.

Travel Vaccines

There are many infections that are rare in the United States and other developed countries but remain common in many parts of the world. To protect yourself and your child while vacationing, everyone should consider these additional vaccines.

Depending on where you are going, the vaccine requirement may be different. The best resource to get the most up-to-date information on travel vaccines is your doctor. In addition, you may consult the CDC website (*www.cdc.gov*) for updated information as well. The following section describes some of the more common travel vaccines you may need before departure.

Typhoid Vaccine

Typhoid fever is a dangerous infection caused by the salmonella bacteria. It kills more than 200,000 people in the world each year, and about 400 American travelers catch the disease per year. Those unfortunate enough to get the infection suffer from high fever and extreme fatigue, and they may develop a rash all over the body. Enlargement of the spleen can also be a problem.

The infection is most common in Southeast Asia, but it is also a threat in Africa, the Caribbean, and Central and South America. The most common way to get the infection is by eating contaminated food. You are likely to get sick from this infection even during relatively short trips (less than a week).

Luckily, the typhoid vaccine is readily available, and it works fairly well (offering 50–80 percent protection from typhoid fever). The vaccine is available orally, and four doses are needed for best protection. The last dose of the vaccine should be taken at least one week prior to departure. The vaccine is quite safe, but it can still cause fever and headache in some individuals (less than 5 percent of the time).

Yellow Fever Vaccine

Yellow fever is caused by a virus that is transmitted to humans from mosquito bites. The infection is most common in parts of Africa and South America. Symptoms of the illness range from mild fever and headache to life-threatening bleeding of internal organs. About half of those with severe bleeding die from the infection.

The yellow fever vaccine is recommended for all travelers older than nine months of age to parts of the world where yellow fever is common. A single dose of the vaccine offers protection for more than ten years.

⚠ Alert

The yellow fever vaccine contains weakened but live viruses. It is not recommended for pregnant women and individuals with severely weakened immune systems, including those with cancer or AIDS.

The yellow fever vaccine has not been implicated in any serious reactions, but mild side effects, including mild headache and muscle ache, may bother some people. Pregnant women and people who are severely allergic to chicken egg should not get this vaccine.

Japanese Encephalitis Vaccine

Japanese encephalitis, as its name suggests, is common in Asia. More than 50,000 people get sick from it each year all over Asia. If you plan to spend some time in Asia, you definitely should protect yourself with this vaccine.

Japanese encephalitis is transmitted by mosquito bites. Stricken individuals develop fever and headache, and they may become disoriented. Serious complications from the infection include coma, paralysis, and death.

Even though the infection is widespread in Asia, not all travelers to Asian countries need to be vaccinated. Transmission of the infection during seasons when the mosquito population is low (from October to April) is uncommon. Consult your doctor or a special travel nurse for up-to-date information on the necessity of the vaccine for your itinerary. Three doses of the vaccine are recommended for travelers. The vaccine is quite safe, but it can cause life-threatening allergic reactions in some individuals.

The Hepatitis A Vaccine

Even though the hepatitis A vaccine is now routinely recommended for children at age one and two years, this recommendation was made relatively recently (2006). This means that many adolescents and adults have not had the hepatitis A vaccine.

The hepatitis A vaccine is recommended for anyone who has not been vaccinated and who is planning to travel to any developed countries. Consult your doctor or a travel nurse to find out whether you should get vaccinated against hepatitis A prior to departure. Even though two doses of the hepatitis A vaccine are recommended, the first dose of the vaccine can offer significant protection against the infection. The second dose of the vaccine is needed to offer lifelong protection.

Recent Changes in the Vaccine Schedule

Several modifications have been made to the childhood immunization schedule since 2007. These changes are made to accommodate the introduction of new vaccines, recent vaccine shortages, and new information about the safety and efficacy of existing vaccines.

The hepatitis A vaccine used to be recommended for children and adults living in parts of the United States that have a large immigrant population. Starting in 2006, the hepatitis A vaccine is now recommended for all children. Previously the hepatitis A vaccine was recommended for children two years and older, but now the lower age limit has been changed to one year. As a result of this recent change, many adolescents and adults are not vaccinated for hepatitis A.

Also in 2006, a second dose of the chickenpox vaccine was recommended. This additional dose is important because many children remain susceptible to chickenpox even after receiving one dose of the chickenpox vaccine. The chickenpox vaccine only works about 85 percent of the time after the first dose, but it works more than 98 percent of the time after the second dose. Since this recommendation was made relatively recently, your child may not have had the second dose of the chickenpox vaccine. Check your child's immunization record or consult your pediatrician to see whether your child still needs a second chickenpox vaccine.

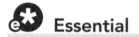 **Essential**

If your child has a weakened immune system, it may be prudent not to skip the final dose of the Hib vaccine because he is more susceptible to this infection. If your child has sickle cell anemia, has had surgery to remove the spleen, or has had organ transplantation, he should get the complete series of the Hib vaccine despite the shortage.

The HPV vaccine was introduced in 2006, and it was incorporated into the childhood immunization schedule in the same year. At this time, this vaccine is not mandatory for school attendance, and many medical offices do not routinely administer this vaccine due to the high cost of immunization (it costs approximately $400 for the three-dose series, including the cost of administration).

The live nasal flu vaccine is now recommended for children down to age two. Previously the lower age limit for this vaccine was five years. Nevertheless, this live flu vaccine is still not recommended for children suffering from wheezing or asthma.

In June of 2009, the CDC announced that the Hib conjugate vaccine shortage was over. However, the shortage that existed previously (from 2007 to 2009) means that your child may not have received the total number of doses of this vaccine. At this time, the CDC does not recommend children returning to the doctor's office to make up for the missing dose.

Other modifications may have occurred to the immunization schedule after this book was published. You should consult your doctor for the most current recommendation.

CHAPTER 7

The Hepatitis B Vaccine

T he hepatitis B vaccine is among the most controversial vaccines because it is often given to babies at birth. In addition, this vaccine used to contain a mercury-based preservative, and many people were concerned about the potential harmful effect of exposure to mercury at such a young age. This chapter will explore the various facets of the controversy and allow you to make an educated decision about this vaccine.

Introduction

Many parents are concerned about the safety of this vaccine because some hepatitis B vaccines contained a mercury-based preservative in the past. However, the mercury preservative has been eliminated from all childhood vaccines, including the hepatitis B vaccine, since 2001. Additional controversy surrounding this vaccine centers on its necessity. Since this is an infection that is primarily transmitted sexually and through intravenous drug use, some parents are reluctant to subject their newborn babies to this vaccine due to the low risk of exposure at that age.

The hepatitis B vaccine is often the first immunization that your baby receives. In most hospitals, this vaccine is given at birth. The rational for administering this vaccine soon after delivery is that if the mother is infected with hepatitis B, she could potentially pass on the infection to the baby during birth. If a baby gets the infection from the mother at the time of birth, a serious infection is more likely to sicken the baby.

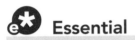 **Essential**

The hepatitis B vaccine is hailed as the first vaccine against cancer because chronic hepatitis B infection is the most common cause of liver cancer. Liver cancer is the most devastating complication resulting from the hepatitis B infection. Around the world, millions die from liver cancer each year.

Since this vaccine only became available recently, many adolescents have not gotten this vaccine during childhood. Check your teen's immunization record to find out whether she still needs to get the hepatitis B series. It takes three shots over the course of six months to get full protection from the infection.

Hepatitis B Infection

Hepatitis B is a unique illness because chronic infection can lead to the development of liver cancer. Even though the majority of people who get this infection ultimately recover, those who are left with a chronic infection are at a high risk of developing liver failure and liver cancer. These serious complications make this infection an important one to prevent.

Most people who catch hepatitis B suffer no outward symptoms. However, the infection can remain dormant or it can lead to chronic liver infection that eventually causes the liver to fail. Some people can suffer jaundice, fatigue, nausea, and other vague symptoms when they first get this infection. Occasionally infected individuals can develop arthritis and a rash from the virus. Most people who harbor the virus have no idea that they are infected.

Even though these infected people feel completely healthy, they can still pass the infection to others.

 Fact

If you get hepatitis B as an adult, you will make a complete recovery more than 95 percent of the time. However, if your baby gets hepatitis B, she will develop liver failure and liver cancer more than 80 percent of the time. The immature immune system makes babies more vulnerable to hepatitis B infection.

Symptoms of Hepatitis B

The symptoms of hepatitis B can often take years to show. In fact, many people who have the disease do not know that they have it. Symptoms can include:

- Extreme fatigue
- Weight loss even though you weren't trying to; general loss of appetite
- Jaundice (the skin or whites of the eyes may turn yellow)
- Nausea
- Vomiting
- Headache
- Excruciating pain in the belly (particularly on the right side where the liver is located)
- Joint pain
- Muscle aches

How Does One Catch It?

The hepatitis B virus is spread by bodily fluids, including blood, semen, vaginal secretion, and saliva. In countries where hepatitis B is common, the infection is frequently passed on from the infected mother to the newborn baby at the time of birth. In most developed countries, this method of transmission is uncommon because most pregnant women are not infected.

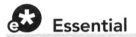 **Essential**

Even though hepatitis B cannot be transmitted via casual contacts (such as kissing), the virus is present in saliva. It can be passed between members of the same household. The exact route of transmission is unclear in this situation.

Nevertheless, hepatitis B still infects many individuals in developed countries because it is sexually transmitted. Being much more contagious than HIV, hepatitis B is a major sexually transmitted disease in the United States. It is especially common among homosexual men.

 Alert

About 30 percent of the people who are infected with hepatitis B have never abused drugs, have had sexual partners who did not have hepatitis B, and have never received a blood transfusion. For these individuals, how they contracted hepatitis B is unknown.

Since the virus is present in the blood, one can acquire this infection from intravenous drug use or through blood transfusion. Despite valiant efforts to screen blood donors for this infection, it is still possible to get this infection from blood transfusion. This explains why hepatitis B infection is more common among those who get frequent blood transfusions (such as patients with hemophilia or sickle cell disease).

How Common Is the Infection?

Worldwide, hepatitis B is a common and serious infection. More than one million people around the world die from liver failure or liver cancer resulting from hepatitis B infection. Fortunately, this infection is rare in the United States and other developed countries. However, due to the large influx of immigration to many countries and the ease of international travel, it is becoming increasingly common, even in developed parts of the world.

 Fact

> About 1.25 million people in the United States have chronic hepatitis B infection, and more than 4,000 people die each year from hepatitis B liver disease, including liver failure and liver cancer.

Since most people who are infected show no symptoms, the only way to find those who are infected is through a blood test. There is no routine screening for hepatitis B, so the number of infections in the general population could actually be higher. Most people infected with hepatitis B have no idea that they carry the infection in their body.

How Serious Is the Infection?

Hepatitis B can cause chronic liver infection that ultimately causes the liver to fail. In addition, chronic liver infection can trigger liver cancer. Both liver failure and liver cancer are difficult to treat, and they are almost inevitably fatal. You do not develop any symptoms of liver cancer until the cancer has spread to the lungs or the brain.

These devastating complications of hepatitis B infection do not usually occur until later in life, when the victim has already had the chance of passing the infection to a spouse and children. Unless the chain of infection is interrupted by prevention, hepatitis B is a curse that gets passed on from one generation to the next. Any child born to an infected mother gets a sentence for early demise at birth.

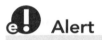 **Alert**

There is a reliable blood test to check for hepatitis B infection, and this test is routinely done in pregnant women. Nevertheless, many women go through pregnancy without prenatal care due to lack of health in- surance, and if these women were infected they would unknowingly pass the infection to their babies.

Is the Infection Treatable?

While there are medications to treat hepatitis B infection, there is no cure. The options are limited, and the treatment does not work well in most cases. These medications are aimed to reduce the chance of liver failure and liver cancer from chronic hepatitis B infection. If the infection is acquired during early childhood, the medications are especially useless.

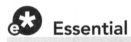 **Essential**

Several new drugs have been approved in the last five years to treat hepatitis B. They work by stopping the virus from reproducing inside the body. They bring new hope to the horizon of hepatitis B treat- ment, but none of them is capable of eradicating the infection.

In most cases, the treatments only postpone the more serious ill- nesses. They simply buy more time for the victim, and they do not offer any real hope for those who already have chronic liver infection.

If a mother infected with hepatitis B is found to have the infection at the time of birth, she can receive immunoglobulin against hepatitis B to reduce the chance of her passing the infection to her baby. This emergency treatment, however, depends on the availability of the immunoglobulin. This treatment is not possible for home deliveries.

Components of the Hepatitis B Vaccine

The hepatitis B vaccine is made from a part of the virus. This is usually synthesized in the laboratory in the test tube, but other parts of the world still manufacture the vaccine from human blood. In the United States, this vaccine is uniformly produced artificially, so there is no possibility of contamination from live virus or other germs. In either case, because the vaccine contains only a part of the actual virus, the vaccine itself cannot cause hepatitis B.

Alert

The hepatitis B vaccine used to contain the mercury-based preservative thimerosal, but this preservative hasn't been added to the vaccine since 2001. Currently no hepatitis B vaccine contains thimerosal as a preservative.

A small amount of aluminum is added to the hepatitis B vaccine because the virus alone does not trigger enough of an immune response to the vaccine. The added aluminum boosts the immune system's reaction to the vaccine, allowing the vaccine to work better. If you are concerned about the presence of aluminum in vaccines, please refer to Chapter 4.

Side Effects of the Hepatitis B Vaccine

The hepatitis B vaccine can cause some soreness and swelling at the site of injection in some children, but the symptoms are more annoying than dangerous. The local reactions usually go away after a day or two.

Anaphylaxis

There are two potentially serious reactions from the hepatitis B vaccine. The first is a life-threatening allergic reaction to the vaccine, and the second is the association between some autoimmune diseases with the vaccine.

One of out every 600,000 times the hepatitis B vaccine is given, someone may experience a severe allergic reaction to the vaccine. This includes swelling of the mouth and throat, wheezing, difficulty breathing, and shock. This is an extremely dangerous reaction that requires emergency medical intervention. Such reaction typically happens shortly after the injection, usually within fifteen minutes.

Alert

Fortunately, the allergic reaction can be reversed with prompt treatment, and death can be prevented. Nevertheless, this is a serious reaction to keep in mind. It is a good idea to stay around the medical facility for twenty minutes after receiving the hepatitis B vaccine.

The Story of Julie

The second type of serious reaction linked to the hepatitis B vaccine is more controversial. So far, the verdict is mixed among vaccine experts. Some studies have demonstrated a temporal relationship between the vaccine and various autoimmune disorders, including Guillain Barré Syndrome.

Julie is a registered nurse who received her first hepatitis B vaccine when she was thirty-seven years old. Three days after she was vaccinated, she developed weakness in her legs and she couldn't walk the next day. She was hospitalized and had a spinal tap. The doctors diagnosed her with Guillain Barré Syndrome, which is a condition that is caused by one's own immune system attacking the nerves in the body. Several vaccines have been linked with this condition, including the hepatitis B vaccine, the flu vaccine, and a type of meningitis vaccine (the meningococcal conjugate vaccine).

The weakness gradually spread to Julie's arms and face, but fortunately she never stopped breathing. She did have difficulty eating and swallowing secondary to the weakness. Her weakness gradually improved, and she left the hospital after two weeks.

It has been two months since Julie got her hepatitis B vaccine, and she is still using crutches to walk. Her life has been drastically altered by what happened, and she worries about her future and whether she will eventually make a full recovery.

The Autoimmune Association

Besides Guillain Barré Syndrome, other autoimmune disorders, including multiple sclerosis and optic neuritis, have been linked to the hepatitis B vaccine. However, it is extremely difficult to either prove or disprove whether there is a causal relationship. The difficulty lies in the fact that these conditions are rare.

Some vaccine experts believe that the hepatitis B vaccine could cause Guillain Barré Syndrome, but other research has refuted this connection. At this time, the best approach is to be aware of the possibility of this serious vaccine reaction and consider the risk of being exposed to hepatitis B at the same time. For some individuals, the risk of contracting the hepatitis B infection far outweighs the risk of developing Guillain Barré Syndrome. You are more likely to catch hepatitis B if you work with patients in the health-care industry or if your work involves close contact with blood products or other bodily secretions. In addition, if you have a condition that requires frequent blood transfusions (such as sickle cell disease or hemophilia), it is a good idea for you to get vaccinated against hepatitis B.

Keep in mind that Guillain Barré Syndrome is quite rare, and many other infections can trigger Guillain Barré Syndrome. It is proven that certain stomach infections can trigger Guillain Barré Syndrome. Finally, most patients with Guillain Barré Syndrome make a full recovery. It may take many months or even years, but permanent disability resulting from Guillain Barré is unusual.

Sudden Infant Death Syndrome

Many parents also report that the hepatitis B vaccine killed their babies. However, when you look at the number of babies who die from sudden infant death syndrome (SIDS) who have never gotten the hepatitis B vaccine and the ones who did, the number is the same. SIDS is the number one cause of death for babies, even before the hepatitis B vaccine was invented. Despite having babies sleeping on their backs instead of their tummies, which has greatly reduced the number of deaths, many babies still die from SIDS today.

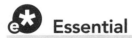 **Essential**

A study in 2008 showed that the use of a ceiling fan or portable fan can significantly reduce the chance of babies dying from SIDS. The theory is that the fan reduces the room temperature, and a hot room poses greater risk for babies who may die from SIDS.

More babies died from SIDS in the days before the hepatitis B vaccine was ever invented than today, and the introduction of hepatitis B vaccine did not lead to an increased number of deaths for babies. It is very unlikely that the hepatitis B vaccine is responsible for SIDS. Some babies inevitably die from SIDS after receiving the hepatitis B vaccine, but these babies would most likely suffer from SIDS whether they received the hepatitis B vaccine or not.

The most important thing you can do as a parent to protect your baby from SIDS is to always place your baby on her back to sleep and use a fan in the room when your baby is sleeping. Avoid putting any pillows, stuffed animals, or loose blankets in the crib. Use a wearable body wrap blanket instead of a loose one to prevent suffocation that can be caused if your baby gets tangled.

CHAPTER 8

The DTaP Vaccine

The DTaP vaccine has been the focus of much debate. It is the vaccine known to trigger seizures and high fever. At the same time, it is also the vaccine that is responsible for protecting children from some of the deadliest infections, including whooping cough and tetanus. Therefore, it is particularly important to learn the risks and benefits of this vaccine.

Introduction

The vaccine against whooping cough, tetanus, and diphtheria is an old vaccine, but the version of the vaccine your child is getting is relatively new. The newer version of this vaccine was introduced in 2000 to reduce side effects resulting from the older vaccine.

The *D* in DTaP represents diphtheria, an infection that is associated with severe cough and seizures. The *T* in DTaP stands for tetanus, which is an infection that is commonly known as lockjaw. The *a* in DTaP was added in 2000 to distinguish the newer version of this vaccine from the older type, which was manufactured differently. Finally, the *P* in DTaP is the pertussis component of the vaccine. Pertussis is also known as whooping cough. All three infections will be described individually in detail in the following sections.

The DTaP vaccine is one of the oldest vaccines. The tetanus vaccine became available in 1924, and the diphtheria vaccine came out in the same year. When these two vaccines were first developed, treatment for these infections was dangerous and frequently unavailable to those who needed them. Due to the effectiveness of these vaccines, you probably never heard of anyone with these conditions. The whooping cough vaccine was invented in 1926, and these three vaccines were combined in the mid-1940s to decrease the number of injections children receive.

This vaccine has undergone much evolution in the past decades, and the reason for the changes is primarily to reduce the side effects associated with this vaccine. The older version of this vaccine, called the DTP vaccine (or the whole-cell DTP vaccine), used to cause fever in children up to half of the time after its administration. In addition, it was associated with swelling of the brain in rare circumstances. It is believed that the way the older vaccine was manufactured was responsible for these side effects. The pertussis component of the older vaccine was made from the entire germ that causes whooping cough, which is why it was called the whole-cell DTP vaccine. The current version of the vaccine was introduced in 2000, and the new DTaP vaccine is manufactured from parts of the pertussis bacteria instead of the entire germ. Since its introduction, it is clear that the chance of having swelling at the injection site, fever, and loss of appetite is much lower than in the past with the older whole-cell vaccine.

Diphtheria

Diphtheria is not a well-known infection. Most people who are not health-care workers probably have never heard of this disease. You might have never heard of this infection because it is now extremely rare. Diphtheria is a serious infection that causes swelling and destruction of the tissues of the throat as well as damage in the heart muscle and the nerves. The bacteria release a poison that kills brain cells and damages nerves throughout the body.

Symptoms of Diphtheria Infection

The early symptoms of diphtheria can be mistaken for a bad sore throat:

- Fever
- Fatigue
- Nausea
- Problems swallowing
- Sore throat
- Swollen glands

But symptoms can then progress further to more serious concerns:

- Vomiting
- Chills
- High fever
- Neck swelling
- Breathing problems

How Does One Catch It?

Diphtheria is a bacterium that only affects humans, so you cannot catch it from your pets. It is passed on from one person to the next from discharge from the nose, eyes, and saliva. Most likely it is transmitted when the sick person coughs violently and sprays his surroundings with the bacteria. It can be also passed on when the sick person wipes his secretions with his hands and then touches another person with the contaminated hands. In rare occasions, diphtheria can also cause skin or eye infections, which spread by direct contact.

How Common Is the Infection?

In the 1920s, diphtheria used to be one of the most common causes of death for children. More than 150,000 people were stricken with diphtheria each year before the vaccine was available. Since the introduction of the vaccine, diphtheria is now extremely rare in the United States and other developed countries. Today, less than five people per year are diagnosed with the infection in the United States. However, in parts of the world where vaccines are not widely available, sporadic outbreaks still occur.

How Serious Is the Infection?

The throat swelling caused by diphtheria is life threatening. The damaged tissues sloughing off the airway can completely block air from entering into the lungs, and the victim suffocates. About 5 to 10 percent of children with diphtheria die from it, but even the survivors suffer permanent heart and nerve damage. The poison released by the bacteria is particularly dangerous. It causes direct damage to the brain and nerves, causing seizures that are difficult to stop.

 Fact

The abnormally severe muscle contraction in tetanus is caused by the poison released by the bacteria. The poison interferes with the communication between nerves and muscles. It prevents the nerves from relaxing the muscles, so the muscles end up in a fixed, contracted state.

Is the Infection Treatable?

Fortunately, this often-deadly infection is treatable. However, antibiotics and antidotes against the poison released must be given promptly. A delay in diagnosis and treatment could result in death, and some may die despite the appropriate treatment. If your child gets infected with diphtheria, he would need to be hospitalized in the intensive care unit for at least two weeks to receive intravenous medications.

Tetanus

Tetanus is most commonly known by the general public as lockjaw. This nickname came from the fact that when a person is stricken by the poison released by this bacteria, every muscle in the body tenses up, including the jaw and facial muscles. Consequently, the mouth is locked in a painful grimace.

The tetanus vaccine stands out among all vaccines because it works better than any vaccines currently available. Historically, it has saved millions of lives and transformed world history. During World War I, before the tetanus vaccine was available, tetanus from injuries was the number one cause of death for soldiers on the battlefield. In contrast, out of 12 million soldiers in World War II, only six died from tetanus. Those who died were later found not to have received the tetanus vaccine.

Symptoms of Tetanus

Symptoms of tetanus include:

- Jaw stiffness
- Difficulty swallowing
- Fever
- Chills
- Sore throat
- Throat spasms
- Stiff arms and legs, general muscle spasms
- Facial muscle spasms
- Back muscle spasms and stiffness
- Difficulty breathing and respiratory spasms
- Paralysis

⊙ Alert

Without proper and timely treatment, tetanus is almost always fatal. The tetanus toxin causes the entire body to tense up, leading to asphyxiation. Diagnosis is often delayed because most doctors do not recognize it due to the rarity of this condition in the United States today.

How Does One Catch It?

The bacteria that causes tetanus is present everywhere. It lives in the soil, and it can be found on any contaminated surface. It also lives inside the guts of people and animals.

The bacteria cannot penetrate normal healthy skin. It can gain access into the body only if there's a cut or wound. You can contract tetanus if you are injured by a dirty object or if your skin is dirty when it is injured. You cannot catch tetanus from another person with tetanus.

⊛ Essential

Contrary to common belief, you do not have to step on a rusty nail to contract tetanus. Any wound that is dirty can result in tetanus, but a deep penetrating injury is especially prone to tetanus infection.

Since the bacteria that causes tetanus is present in the intestines of people and animals, animal and human bites are common sources of tetanus infection. Also, in developing countries, newborn babies frequently die from tetanus because mothers are often not adequately immunized and dirty instruments are used to cut the umbilical cord at birth.

How Common Is the Infection?

In the United States, tetanus has become extremely rare. In the past decade, less than fifty cases of tetanus have been reported a year in this country. However, it is still a common problem worldwide, especially in parts of the world where the health-care system is deficient.

How Serious Is the Infection?

Tetanus is a life-threatening infection. The poison released by the bacterium causes simultaneous contraction of all the muscles in the body, including the muscles that allow you to breath. If the spasm lasts too long, death from asphyxiation results.

Is the Infection Treatable?

Antidote for the tetanus poison must be given promptly if the infection is likely. In addition to antibiotics, a booster vaccine should be given whenever tetanus is suspected. If the treatment is delayed, death can result despite the proper management. Thoroughly cleaning any wound is another way to reduce the chance of catching this infection.

Pertussis

Pertussis is commonly called whooping cough. The name is derived from the sound of the person quickly sucking in air—the "whoop"—after a violent bout of coughing. The primary symptom of the infection is coughing, which can be quite prolonged. It is not uncommon for the cough to last more than two months. The cough is typically so severe that vomiting often occurs after the violent coughing spells. People with whooping cough usually have no fever or only have very slight fever.

Symptoms of Whooping Cough

The first stages of pertussis can have the following symptoms:

- Running nose
- Sneezing
- Cough similar to common cold

Gradually the symptoms will worsen and include:

- Coughing spells (can last more than one minute)
- Turning blue or red from lack of oxygen during coughing
- Vomiting following a coughing attack

How Does One Catch It?

The infection is passed on from one person to another through the air. The violent cough sprays infected droplets of saliva into the air, and another person can inhale the germ through the nose. Only humans can get whooping cough, so you cannot make your pets sick (and vice versa).

🅔❗ Alert

Pertussis is a highly contagious illness. If someone at your house has whooping cough, there is a 90 percent chance that everyone in the household will come down with whooping cough if their immunization is not up to date.

Older children and adults are the most common sources of infection for babies. Since older children and adults frequently have milder coughs, many chronic coughs are not recognized as whooping cough and they remain untreated.

How Common Is the Infection?

Whooping cough outbreaks occur in three- to five-year cycles. It is still quite common, even in developed nations, including the United States. Each year, between 600,000 and

900,000 people are diagnosed with whooping cough in the United States.

Recently, more and more parents are electing not to immunize their children because of concerns about the safety of this vaccine. Consequently, there is an increasing number of outbreaks in the community.

How Serious Is the Infection?

Whooping cough is usually not life threatening for adolescents and adults. The cough can be quite uncomfortable and violent. Hospitalization for adults is rare for this infection.

However, if a baby catches whooping cough, it is usually a serious ordeal. The coughing can be so violent that it interferes with the baby's breathing, and babies less than six months old often do not have the "whoop" after the bout of coughing. Affected infants frequently stop breathing momentarily and turn blue. Frequent cough attacks can result in seizure and permanent brain damage due to lack of oxygen to the brain. Premature babies are at even higher risk, and fatality is not uncommon.

 Fact

Babies less than six months old are most likely to die from whooping cough. As a child grows older, her breathing is less likely to be affected by whooping cough, but she can still spread the illness to others.

Is the Infection Treatable?

The infection itself is not treatable once the coughing starts, but doctors often prescribe antibiotics once the diagnosis is confirmed because treatment makes it less likely for the patient to pass the infection to other people. The antibiotic does not alleviate the cough or shorten the duration of the illness.

While the infection itself cannot be treated, babies with whooping cough are usually hospitalized to monitor their breathing. If the baby stops breathing from the severe cough, a breathing machine is necessary to force air into the baby's lungs. Many babies with whooping cough are cared for in the intensive care unit.

Alert

The antibiotic used to treat whooping cough is called erythromycin. When this antibiotic is given to babies less than six weeks of age, it can cause intestinal blockage that requires surgery.

Components of the DTaP Vaccine

The DTaP vaccine is a combination vaccine. It contains a weakened toxin from the diphtheria bacterium, a weakened toxin from the tetanus bacterium, and modified proteins from the whooping cough bacterium.

 Fact

The obsolete DTP vaccine used to contain killed whooping cough germs. The new DTaP vaccine does not contain any live or dead germs, unlike the older DTP vaccine. Therefore, this vaccine cannot cause an infection.

The toxins in the DTaP vaccine are weakened after soaking for prolonged period of time in formaldehyde, which renders the toxins harmless. The toxins are chemically altered in the process so that they no longer make people sick, but they can still alert the immune system and generate a "memory" response for the immune system. Because of the vaccine's manufacturing process, a small amount of formaldehyde is present in the vaccine.

In addition, a small amount of aluminum is added to the vaccine to make the vaccine work better. The aluminum is responsible for some of the redness and pain at the site of injection. However, the amount is very small. If you are concerned about the aluminum content in vaccines, please refer to Chapter 4 on vaccine safety.

Side Effects of the DTaP Vaccine

The DTP vaccine is notorious because it is associated with the most side effects. It is also the vaccine that single-handedly triggered the modern antivaccine movement. With the advent of the newer DTaP vaccine, most of the side effects linked to the older vaccine are much milder and occur with lower frequency.

Question

If my baby developed a fever after the DTaP vaccine, is it safe for him to get the same vaccine in the future?
Children who experience these common reactions (fever, loss of appetite, crying) can still receive the DTaP vaccine in the future. Even though similar reactions may occur with future vaccination, they are quite harmless.

The most common side effect is tenderness at the site of injection. This can last for more than three days. In addition, swelling and redness over a large area of the skin where the injection was given can last up to two weeks. Even though these side effects are common, parents tend not to worry much about these reactions because they are so mild and do not have any lasting effect.

Fever is another common side effect, which occurs in approximately 20 to 25 percent of the children receiving this vaccine. Loss of appetite and irritability are also common side effects. Even though these reactions are common, they go away in a few days and do not cause any permanent problems.

Some of the more serious reactions to the DTaP vaccine include seizures and unusually prolonged crying. These reactions have been proven to occur after the administration of the DTaP vaccine, and most experts agree that the vaccine is responsible for these reactions. Fortunately, these reactions rarely occur. Only about 1 in 14,000 children develops seizures, and 1 in 1,000 children may have excessive crying. Even though these reactions are scary and need a thorough medical investigation after they occur, they do not lead to permanent problems with the brain.

The heart of controversy surrounding the DTaP vaccine is that it has been linked to serious but rare problems. In particular, the developments of seizures and swelling in the brain have been implicated with the older DTP vaccine. The biggest controversy is whether the current DTaP vaccine can cause permanent brain damage.

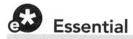 **Essential**

Most of the studies done about the safety of the whooping cough vaccine were based on the older DTP vaccine that is no longer used. Less is known about the current DTaP acellular vaccine, but most experts and doctors agree that the new DTaP vaccine causes significantly less side effects than the old DTP vaccine.

In the 1990s, a flurry of research activities took place to answer this specific question. At the time, only the older whole-cell DTP vaccine was being used. A British study demonstrated that the link between the old DTP vaccine and brain damage is definitely possible, and such reaction could affect 1 in 140,000 children receiving the DTP vaccine. Subsequent studies in Great Britain as well as the United States have put the original British study in doubt. Nevertheless, no study can completely refute any association between the old DTP vaccine and permanent brain damage.

If you are more confused about the relationship between the DTaP vaccine and brain damage after reading this, you are not alone. Even experts cannot agree whether the DTaP vaccine can cause brain damage. One thing that everyone can agree on is that if such a devastating side effect could be caused by the DTaP vaccine, it is extremely rare. Most doctors believe that the frequency of such reaction is on the order of one in a million.

It is probably impossible to ever prove or disprove a causal relationship between the DTaP vaccine and brain damage. The difficulty for such research is that brain damage is so rare. Intuitively, you can imagine that if the DTaP vaccine causes brain damage in a majority of children, there wouldn't be any healthy children by now.

Alert

If your child has existing neurologic problems, such as recurrent seizures or severe developmental delay, talk to your pediatrician about the risk of the DTaP vaccine. Certain individuals are more susceptible to seizures triggered by the vaccine. The doctor may decide to postpone the DTaP vaccine or forgo it altogether.

On the other hand, the possibility that DTaP vaccine causes brain damage certainly exists, but there are ways to avoid such reaction. Children with existing brain damage or deteriorating neurological disorders should be exempt from the DTaP vaccine, and children with severe seizures should not receive the DTaP vaccine until their seizures are brought under control.

Tdap Booster

The Tdap booster shot is a relatively new vaccine. It replaced the older tetanus booster shot (Td) for adolescents and adults, which was recommended for children older than eleven years of age and adults. This vaccine contains the same amount of tetanus component as the childhood DTaP vaccine, but it contains less diphtheria and whooping cough components. Consequently, the Tdap vaccine is less likely to cause fever and local swelling of the skin.

🔔 Alert

If you are concerned about thimerosal, the new Tdap vaccine does not contain any thimerosal. The Tdap vaccine is manufactured differently than the older Td tetanus booster, which did contain thimerosal.

The Tdap booster functions similarly to the DTaP vaccine for children. Receiving this vaccine reminds one's immune system about the tetanus, diphtheria, and whooping cough infection. This vaccine is unique because it is recommended for all adults every ten years, and it has no upper limit age range. You should check with your doctor to see whether you are due for a Tdap booster. Remember, most babies catch whooping cough from family members, primarily older children and adults. Being up to date on the whooping cough shot not only protects you, but it protects your children from whooping cough.

CHAPTER 9

The Polio Vaccine

T he polio vaccine is controversial not because of its side effects but because some people question whether this vaccine is even necessary in this country anymore. There hasn't been a case of paralytic polio in the United States since 1993, and it has become extinct in all developed countries. This chapter presents the background of the polio infection and the pros and cons of the polio vaccine.

Introduction

Polio has not always been a serious and life-threatening infection. The irony is that it is a disease that has gotten worse with improved sanitation. Prior to the 1920s, polio paralysis was relatively rare. Starting in the 1930s, however, polio started to become a major threat to the newly industrialized America. Major outbreaks that affected thousands and left whole communities paralyzed spread fear throughout this country in the 1950s. Franklin D. Roosevelt pioneered government programs to fund polio research and the development of polio vaccine.

When the world was dirtier and people were frequently exposed to foods contaminated with human feces, polio frequently infected people when they were still very young. When babies get polio, they usually do not suffer the devastating paralytic complication, but they do become permanently immune to polio for the rest of their lives. When older children and adults catch the infection, however, the chance of them being paralyzed is much higher.

As living standards improved, most children did not have the opportunity to be infected when they were young because the environment around them was much cleaner. But if they caught the infection at an older age, they were more likely to suffer the severe neurological problems caused by polio. This is clearly a disease that was made more serious due to improvements in living conditions.

e✱ Essential

The March of Dimes was a foundation started by Roosevelt in the 1930s to fight polio. The foundation has since evolved into an organization to prevent premature birth and promote healthy pregnancy.

Consequently, as urbanization continues, the polio epidemic becomes a greater threat. During an outbreak in 1952, 3,145 people died from polio, and more than 20,000 people became permanently paralyzed from the infection. Worst of all, it is an infection that affects the poor as well as the rich and famous. Being socially privileged did not lend any protection against this scourge. There was no treatment for polio except the iron lung, which only provided supportive care during the period of the most severe paralysis.

The polio vaccine has been controversial for another reason. Prior to 2000, there were two types of polio vaccines—one containing a live but weakened virus, and another containing killed virus. The live polio vaccine is no longer given today because the vaccine could actually cause paralysis in rare circumstances (about 1 in 2 million doses). It was an accepted risk for vaccination because the risk was so much smaller than catching polio itself. However, by the early 1990s, polio had become so rare in the United States and other developed nations that the majority of the people suffering from polio paralysis actually got polio from the live polio vaccine. By that time, it did not make sense to continue using the live polio vaccine. Only the killed polio vaccine is available in the United States today.

 Alert

With the live polio vaccine, the risk of becoming paralyzed as a vaccine side effect was 1 in 2.4 million. It was a very small risk, but it was nevertheless present. It is the reason why the live polio vaccine is no longer used.

Polio Infection

When you think of polio, the iron lung may come to mind. Perhaps the image of a wheelchair-bound Franklin D. Roosevelt pops into your consciousness. It is unlikely that you know anyone who is personally affected by polio today, even though there remains a fairly large group of people in the United States who survived polio but are still struggling with the disabilities polio inflicted on them when they were younger.

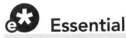 **Essential**

Even though there has not been a new diagnosis of polio for decades in this country, there are still over 400,000 Americans who are disabled as a result of the polio infection. Polio causes permanent paralysis, and its legacy lives on in these people who contracted the disease long ago.

Polio is caused by a virus that only affects humans. This is the reason why it is possible to devise a vaccine that could potentially wipe this disease from the face of this planet. The story behind the development of the polio vaccine is full of intrigue and espionage that is worthy of a full-length book in its own right, and the two scientists who led the effort to invent the polio vaccine became national heroes. They are so famous that the vaccines used today still bear their names—the Salk vaccine and the Sabin vaccine.

✅ Fact

The Salk Institute for Biological Studies in San Diego remains a leader in the scientific community and plays an important role in the advancement of medical research today. The institute now focuses on a variety of biological and medical research.

Symptoms of Polio

Nonparalytic polio has the following symptoms:

- Fever
- Sore throat
- Fatigue
- Back pain and stiffness
- Neck pain and stiffness
- Muscle spasms

Paralytic polio starts with these same symptoms but the individual soon develops:

- Loss of reflexes
- Severe muscle spasms or aches
- Loose and floppy limbs
- Sudden paralysis in either the spinal cord (affecting the muscles that control breathing and the arms and the legs), the brainstream (affecting the cranial nerves that control

your ability to see, speak, hear, taste, and swallow, as well as those that send messages to you heart, intestines, and lungs), or a combination of the two (resulting in paralysis of the arms and legs as well as affecting breathing, swallowing, and heart function)

Post-polio syndrome affects some who have recovered from polio and includes symptoms such as:

- Progressive muscle and joint weakness
- Breathing of swallowing problems
- Muscle atrophy
- General fatigue and exhaustion

How Does One Catch It?

Polio is most often transmitted by eating or drinking contaminated food or water. The virus is passed in the feces of an infected person. If the water supply is contaminated with human excrement, it will act as a reservoir for future infections.

Improving sanitation on a large scale has failed to eradicate this infection in certain parts of the world where living standards are poor. The only hope of getting rid of this disease once and for all is through a comprehensive childhood vaccination program in those remaining countries that harbor the polio virus.

How Common Is the Infection?

Polio is now nonexistent in the United States. The last person diagnosed with paralytic polio in this country got sick in 1979. However, there are still many pockets in the world where polio thrives.

The largest pockets of polio infection remaining in the world are located in India and Nigeria. However, many other countries, such as Afghanistan, Pakistan, Angola, and Chad, continue to harbor hot zones for potential outbreaks. In 2008, over 1,000 people around the globe came down with polio, and the trend is getting worse because there were almost three times as many cases in 2008 compared to 2007.

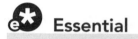 **Essential**

A national Peace Day is scheduled in parts of the world where armed conflicts rampage the country and prevent effective childhood immunization. On Peace Day, both sides of the confrontation lay down their arms and allow children to safely venture into medical clinics to get vaccinated against polio.

Even though the Americans have won the battle against polio, the global fight is losing ground. With international travel, the risk of a future outbreak in the United States remains very real.

How Serious Is the Infection?

Even though most children recover completely from polio without suffering any paralysis, those who do have nerve damage usually experience some degree of permanent disabilities. The virus attacks the nervous system directly, causing irreparable destruction to the spine and the brain. If the spinal cord is seriously damaged, the nerves that control breathing could stop functioning, and asphyxiation will ensue.

Is the Infection Treatable?

There is no medication to treat polio infection. Once paralysis starts, there is no effective way to stop the process. Doctors may insert a breathing tube into your child's lungs to pump oxygen into the body when the nerves that control breathing are damaged.

Historically, it was done with the iron lung because mechanical ventilator technology was primitive and the breathing tube cannot remain in the lungs for long periods of time.

Currently, if paralysis occurs, a portable breathing machine is available to deliver oxygen to the lungs through a tracheostomy (a hole cut through the neck to allow the breathing machine to be connected to the airway).

Components of the Polio Vaccine

The killed polio vaccine is made from virus grown in monkey kidney cells and cultured in bovine blood. The live virus is then killed by the chemical formaldehyde. The viral particles subsequently undergo many rounds of purification to filter out the formaldehyde and other organic components, and the vaccine is preserved with an alcohol: 2-phenoxyethanol. Two antibiotics—streptomycin and neomycin—are added in the vaccine during storage and transport to prevent bacterial contamination of the vaccine. The vaccine does not contain the mercury-based preservative thimerosal. The oral live polio vaccine is no longer used in the United States.

 Alert

If your child is allergic to the antibiotics streptomycin and neomycin (common ingredients in antibiotic ear drops), your child may not be able to receive the killed polio vaccine. Talk to your pediatrician to find out whether this may be a problem for your child.

Side Effects of the Polio Vaccine

The polio vaccine that is being used today is quite safe. It is made from killed polio virus, and there is no live virus in any of the vaccines. It is impossible to contract polio from this vaccine. The vaccine-induced paralysis associated with the live polio vaccine is a concern of the past because the live polio vaccine is no longer used in the United States.

Common Mild Reactions

Common mild reactions can include a sore spot on his arm where your child received the polio injection, but often there will be no fever or rash from the injection. The soreness should resolve in less than two days.

Possible Allergic Reaction

Since the killed polio vaccine is prepared with a cell culture that is treated with antibiotics, the vaccine contains a trace amount of antibiotics—streptomycin, neomycin, and polymyxin B—that remains in the final product. These antibiotics are similar to the ones in the popular triple antibiotic ointment applied to cuts and scrapes (such as Neosporin).

 Fact

Today's polio vaccine no longer contains SV40. Since the 1990s, a new method of vaccine production obviates any possibility of viral contamination in today's polio vaccines.

If your child is allergic to these antibiotics, a life-threatening reaction may occur that includes hives, difficulty breathing, and wheezing. This allergic reaction is very rare, estimated to occur less than one in a million doses.

The SV40 Controversy

Today's polio vaccine is largely out of the limelight for its safety concerns. The main argument against polio vaccination is whether it is still necessary. However, this has not always been the case.

In the 1960s, the safety of the polio vaccine was hotly debated because a new virus was found to have contaminated over 10 million doses of the early polio vaccine.

When the killed polio vaccine was first invented (the Salk polio vaccine), scientists did not know much about viruses. The technology to detect viruses had not yet been invented. Between 1955 and 1961, vaccine manufacturers made polio vaccines using kidney tissues from rhesus monkeys. During the production process, the polio virus grew along side of other viruses present in monkeys. It was originally believed that during the process when the polio virus was killed, these other types of viruses perished as well. Scientists later ascertained that it was not the case.

One type of virus in particular has since come under scrutiny. Dr. Bernice Eddy of the National Institute of Health isolated a virus called SV40 (simian virus 40) in 1961 in the laboratory. She was surprised to learn that if she injected this virus into hamsters, all the hamsters developed tumors. Because of that finding, the government implemented new regulations to eliminate all traces of SV40 from future polio vaccines. However, there was not a recall, and additional doses of the contaminated polio vaccines were administered to children until 1963.

Alert

The injectable form of the polio vaccine (the Salk vaccine) was the primary source of SV40 contamination. About 10 million contaminated doses were given between 1955 and 1961. The oral polio vaccine (the Sabin vaccine) was mostly free of this virus, and it is estimated that about 10,000 contaminated oral polio vaccines were administered.

The ongoing controversy is whether SV40 can trigger cancer in humans. It is known that SV40 can cause cancer in a variety of animals, including guinea pigs, hamsters, and mice. In humans, the virus has been isolated from certain types of tumor cells, including a rare type of lung cancer called mesothelioma, a brain tumor (ependymoma), cancer of the bone (osteosarcoma), and certain types of lymphoma (non-Hodgkin's). Whether some of these cancers are caused by SV40 is not clear. Even though the virus was isolated from some of the tumor cells, many people with these cancers have no evidence that they were ever infected by SV40. The research is ongoing to investigate the possible link between this virus and cancer. However, when looking back to those who were exposed to this virus from the contaminated polio vaccine, there is no increased risk of cancer in this population.

CHAPTER 10

The Hib Vaccine

The Hib vaccine is perhaps one of the least controversial vaccines today. This vaccine worked incredibly well right from the moment it was invented, virtually eliminating a devastating brain infection in children. This vaccine only has mild reactions; the only concern about this vaccine was that at one point it used to contain the preservative thimerosal. But thimerosal has been removed from this and all other pediatric vaccines.

Introduction

The Hib vaccine is relatively new, especially compared to the ancient smallpox vaccine. It was first available in 1990, and now three manufacturers produce this vaccine. Depending on the formulation, this vaccine is given either in three or four doses. All formulations of this vaccine work equally well, and they also share the same side effects.

Sometimes the Hib vaccine is combined with other vaccines and given as a single injection instead of two separate injections. The two vaccines that are sometimes combined with the Hib vaccine are the hepatitis B vaccine and the DTaP vaccine. When the vaccines are combined, the potential side effects from the other vaccine can manifest as well.

😯 Alert

Due to the high demand for this vaccine, there have been frequent nationwide shortages in recent years. Your pediatrician may not be able to provide all doses of this vaccine for your child. Talk to your doctor to find out whether your baby missed this vaccine due to the shortage.

The Hib vaccine works extremely well, yet it is still possible to become ill with the Hib infection after receiving the vaccine. It may take more than two weeks after immunization for the body to generate enough immune response to protect your baby against the Hib infection. During this vulnerable period of time, your child is susceptible to the devastating effect of the Hib infection. In addition, this vaccine needs several boosters to work optimally; there is only moderate protection after a single first dose. Subsequent injections boost the immune system further and offer much better protection.

😊 Essential

An earlier version of the Hib vaccine, called the polysaccharide vaccine, first became available in 1985, but it was discontinued because it did not work very well, especially in babies less than a year old. The current version of the Hib vaccine is completely redesigned, and it has proven to work extremely well, even in babies.

Keep in mind that the Hib bacterium is not the only germ that causes meningitis in children. Many other bacteria, including the pneumococcus bacterium and the meningococcus bacterium, are also common causes of meningitis. Fortunately, there are vaccines for both of these bacteria.

Hib Infection

Hib is the shortened version of *Haemophilus influenza* type b. This is a type of bacteria that can cause a serious brain infection in children called meningitis. This bacterium can also cause a life-threatening throat infection, called epiglottitis, and it sometimes causes bone and joint infections as well.

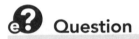 **Question**

Does the Hib bacterium cause the flu?
Even though it has "influenza" in its name, this bacterium has nothing to do with the flu. The flu is caused by a virus, and these two bugs really have nothing in common. Consequently, if your child received the flu shot, she is not protected from this bacterium.

The Hib bacterium used to cause one of the most dreaded childhood infections. A brain infection from this bacterium is extremely dangerous. Even if the infection does not kill your child, it may leave him with permanent hearing loss, mental retardation, or blindness. In addition to brain infection, the Hib bacterium can also cause a life-threatening throat infection that causes the throat to rapidly swell up and cut off the oxygen supply from the body. Less commonly, Hib can also cause infections of the bones and joints. These infections are not as dangerous as the brain or throat infection, but they may cause permanent damage to the bones or joints. Occasionally, the Hib bacterium can also cause pneumonia.

Symptoms of Hib Infection
Symptoms of Hib include:

- High fever
- Irritability
- Weakness

- Vomitting
- Neck stiffness
- Headache
- Swelling in the throat
- Swelling in the brain
- Pneumonia
- Middle ear infection

One out of twenty children with brain infection caused by Hib will die, and many more will be left with more serious disabilities, including blindness, mental retardation, or seizure disorder.

How Does One Catch It?

The Hib infection is highly contagious. It is transmitted from one person to the next by air or direct contact. When one person with the Hib infection coughs or sneezes, the germ is sprayed into the air and another person in close proximity can inhale the bacteria into the body. Surface contamination by the secretions of a sick person can also serve as a way for this infection to spread. Children living in the same household are especially likely to pass the infection around, but it can be transmitted in the school setting as well.

 Fact

The Hib infection is so contagious that if more than one child is diagnosed with the infection, the entire school—including all the students, the teachers, and staff members—needs to take antibiotics so that a massive outbreak will not start.

When patients are hospitalized with the Hib infection, they are not permitted to venture out of their hospital room to protect other patients and health-care workers from this infection. A strict quarantine is necessary to prevent infecting the entire hospital with this dangerous germ.

There is no way to protect your child from the Hib infection 100 percent of the time. Your child is especially at risk for catching this infection if she goes to school or daycare. Breast-feeding exclusively for the first year can confer significant protection against this infection. If you are unable to breast-feed exclusively for at least twelve months, your child should definitely get vaccinated against the Hib bacterium.

How Common Is the Infection?

Before the Hib vaccine was invented, Hib infection used to be the most common cause of bacterial meningitis in children. Each year, 15,000 children came down with meningitis caused by Hib, and 400 to 500 of them died from the infection. More children became mentally retarded from this infection than from any other reason in the United States.

 Alert

Even though this vaccine is extremely safe, fewer and fewer babies are getting this vaccine because of shortage and parental concern with vaccines in general. When the population becomes more susceptible to this infection, the Hib bacterium will make a comeback.

This vaccine became available in 1990, and the number of infections caused by Hib plummeted. Hib meningitis is now a relatively rare infection. In 2002, less than 200 cases of Hib infections were reported to the CDC. Most new doctors trained after 1990 have never seen a brain infection caused by Hib. This could potentially be a problem if Hib infections were to become common again in the future, because most doctors would not be able to recognize this infection, and treatment delay could be a real problem.

How Serious Is the Infection?

Meningitis caused by Hib can be devastating. Five percent of children with brain infection will die despite appropriate antibiotic treatment, and many among the survivors will be left with permanent disabilities, including deafness and mental retardation.

The throat infection caused by Hib is almost as bad as the brain infection. The infection causes rapid swelling of the throat, and doctors frequently need to insert a tube directly into the lungs of these children to prevent suffocation.

Hib can also cause bone and joint infections in children. Even though these types of infections are not as deadly, the bacteria can cause the infected bones and joints to be destroyed and permanently cripple these children. What makes bone infections more difficult to manage is that the infections usually need to be treated with intravenous antibiotics for more than six weeks. Prolonged hospitalization followed by a protracted recovery is the norm for these types of infections.

Is the Infection Treatable?

There are many types of antibiotics that can be used to treat Hib infections, but due to the aggressive nature of the Hib bacterium, children die despite receiving the proper treatment. In addition, if the infection was not diagnosed immediately, the chance of serious complications from the infection is even greater.

Children with Hib infections are often extremely ill, requiring additional support with a breathing machine, oxygen, tube-feeding through the nose, and other additional intensive care support. Medications to reduce the swelling of the brain may be employed to prevent permanent brain damage secondary to the infection.

Components of the Hib Vaccine

The Hib vaccine contains chemicals from the outer covering of the Hib bacterium. Because these chemicals by themselves do not trigger the immune system to generate a response against the bacterium, parts of other bacteria are added to the vaccine to make it work better. In addition, a small amount of aluminum is added to the vaccine to further boost the immune system and enhance the effect of the vaccine. The concern about the aluminum additive is addressed in Chapter 4.

There are a total of five types of Hib vaccines on the market now. Three of them contain just the single Hib vaccine, and two others are combination vaccines. All Hib vaccines are made from a chemical found on the outer coating of the Hib bacterium. This chemical is called polyribosylribitol phosphate, or PRP. This chemical is a type of sugar, but it's not the same as the table sugar you are familiar with. This type of sugar is only found in the Hib bacteria, and it probably does not taste sweet.

Essential

These different types of Hib vaccines have different recommended doses. Ask your doctor to find out how many doses are needed and when they are supposed to be given. When one type is unavailable, the other type may be substituted during time of vaccine shortage.

The PRP component of the vaccine is always chemically connected to a piece of protein because the PRP component alone does not trigger a good immune response, and the Hib vaccine would not work without this additional piece of protein. There are three types of proteins that the PRP component is connected with. The PRP-OMP Hib vaccine is connected to the outer membrane protein of another bacterium called *Neisseria meningitides*. The PRP-T Hib vaccine is connected to a protein made by the tetanus bacterium. The HbOC Hib vaccine is connected to a protein made by the diphtheria bacterium.

The only purpose of the protein components in the various Hib vaccines is to alert the immune system to the presence of the PRP component of the Hib vaccine. You can think of the PRP component of the vaccine as a mug shot of the Hib bacterium, and the protein component of the vaccine is a big spotlight shining directly on the mug shot so that your child's immune system will not miss the mug shot. These additional proteins are not harmful; they are incapable of causing infection.

Beside the PRP and the protein components, all the Hib vaccines also contain a trace of aluminum. The aluminum is necessary because it further draws the attention of the immune system to the part of the body where the vaccine is injected and makes sure that the body does not overlook the mug shot of the bacterium. You can compare the role of the aluminum as sounding an alarm. After the injection is given, both the protein component of the vaccine and the aluminum help draw the attention of the immune system to ensure that the body's defense system takes a good look at the Hib bacterium and remembers it. The next time the real Hib germ tries to invade the body, an attack against it can be quickly mounted and the Hib will have no chance of establishing a successful invasion.

In the past, one form of the Hib vaccine used to contain the preservative thimerosal. However, the Hib vaccine that used to have thimerosal has been thimerosal-free since August 1999. The Hib vaccines made by other manufacturers never contained the thimerosal preservative.

Side Effects of the Hib Vaccine

The Hib vaccine has not been associated with any serious side effects. The vaccine does not contain any live bacterium, therefore it cannot cause an actual infection. It has not been blamed for the autism epidemic, since the epidemic was already rampant before this vaccine was invented.

 Fact

The Hib vaccine is special compared to other vaccines because the immunity generated after the vaccine is actually better than the immunity generated naturally after a Hib infection. In other words, it is possible for your child to get Hib infections over and over again if your child is not vaccinated.

Most frequently, the vaccine can result in redness and pain at the site where the vaccine was injected into the skin. This is not the result of an infection but of skin irritation to the chemicals in the vaccine. This skin reaction is fairly mild, and it does not require any medical treatment. Nevertheless, this skin reaction is common, and it affects about one in four children after being vaccinated.

 Alert

If a fever lasts for more than three days following the Hib vaccine, it is probably not the result of the vaccine. You should bring your child to his pediatrician right away to make sure that he does not have an unrelated infection.

Less commonly, children may develop a mild fever after getting this vaccine. Only about 2 percent of children experience this side effect. Even though a fever may cause more concern, any fever reducer, including acetaminophen (Tylenol) or ibuprofen (Motrin), will bring the temperature down quickly. If fever occurs, it starts within twenty-four hours after the vaccination and does not last for more than three days following the vaccine. Beside the over-the-counter fever reducers and other cooling measures, no additional treatment is necessary for the fever.

Aside from these relatively harmless reactions, no other side effects have been attributed to the Hib vaccine. It would be wonderful if all vaccines were this benign, but this is not the case—at least not yet.

CHAPTER 11

The Pneumococcal Vaccine

The pneumococcal vaccine is one of the newer additions to the list of childhood vaccines. In many ways, this vaccine is closely related to the Hib vaccine. However, there are some notable differences between these two infections and vaccines. This chapter will explore these differences and the similarities.

Introduction

Since the pneumococcus bacterium causes so many common infections in children and adults, scientists have long been laboring to come up with a vaccine against this bug. As a result of this prolonged effort at inventing a vaccine against pneumococcus, there are two types of pneumococcal vaccine today. The first type is called the pneumococcal polysaccharide vaccine, and the second type is called the pneumococcal conjugate vaccine.

The polysaccharide vaccine first became available in 1979, and it is only recommended for individuals whose immune system is weakened. The polysaccharide vaccine was not given to babies because this vaccine does not work for children less than two years old. Because the immune system for children younger than two years is still immature, the polysaccharide vaccine does not trigger the immune response necessary for this vaccine to work.

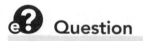 **Essential**

The pneumococcal polysaccharide vaccine is recommended for individuals with sickle cell disease, those without a spleen, people with kidney or liver failure, children who had organ transplantation or undergoing chemotherapy, individuals who are HIV-positive, and senior citizens living in group homes.

Due to this shortcoming, another pneumococcal vaccine was developed. In 2000, a new type of pneumococcal vaccine, called the conjugate pneumococcal vaccine, became available. The conjugate vaccine is made differently than the polysaccharide vaccine, and the conjugate vaccine works well to protect even young babies.

Question

Does my child need both the polysaccharide vaccine and the conjugate vaccine, or are they mutually exclusive?
Even though both the polysaccharide vaccine and the conjugate vaccine protect people from pneumococcal infection, they are designed differently and serve different functions. Some people may need both types of pneumococcal vaccines to protect them from infections.

The polysaccharide pneumococcal vaccine is sometimes known as the "pneumonia" vaccine, because it helps to prevent pneumonia caused by the pneumococcus bacterium. This is a vaccine that is recommended universally for individuals older than sixty-five years and for people with a weak immune system. People with chronic heart, lung, kidney, or liver diseases have a weakened immune system, and they are candidates for the polysaccharide vaccine. In addition, people with diabetes, HIV, cancer, or sickle cell disease should get this vaccine as well. Finally, people without a working spleen should receive this vaccine because the spleen plays an important role in fighting off infection caused by certain types of bacteria, including the pneumococcus bacterium.

On the other hand, the pneumococcal conjugate vaccine is quite similar to the Hib vaccine because they are both recommended for all babies, and they work well in infants younger than two years. Babies who have a problem with their immune system may need to get both the polysaccharide vaccine and the conjugate vaccine. The conjugate vaccine is given first, because the polysaccharide vaccine does not work for children until they are older than two years.

One of the initial concerns about the use of pneumococcal vaccine was that the vaccine could encourage other types of pneumococcus bacterium that are not covered by the vaccine to flourish. Since both types of vaccines only cover a fraction of the total number of types of pneumococci bacteria, doctors have found that other types of pneumococcus bacterium that are not protected by the vaccine are increasingly causing more serious infections. In other words, since the vaccine is designed to target certain types of pneumococcus, other types are taking on the role of triggering infections.

This changing trend means that sooner or later, the usefulness of the pneumococcal vaccines would decrease unless the composition of the vaccine is altered to follow a moving target.

So far, the current pneumococcal vaccine still works quite well for the existing strains of the pneumococcus bacterium. When other strains of pneumococcus not covered by the vaccine start to cause more infections, the vaccines will need to be modified to accommodate the shifting demographics of the pneumococcus bacterium.

Pneumococcal Infection

The pneumococcus bacterium is ubiquitous. It lives in many people's noses and mouths without causing problems to these people. However, these individuals can still pass this bacterium to others and make other people sick. This bacterium causes more ear infections and pneumonia in young children than any other type of bacteria. In addition to these relatively mild infections, pneumococcus can also cause serious infections, such as meningitis and blood infections.

⊕! Alert

The Hib conjugate vaccine was invented before the pneumococcal conjugate vaccine. Since the Hib vaccine worked so well and virtually eliminated Hib meningitis, the pneumococcus bacterium has replaced Hib as the leading cause of bacterial meningitis today.

There are ninety types of pneumococci bacteria. Even though all of them belong to the same kind of bacterium, each type has its own distinct characteristics. You can think of each type as a distinct country in the world. Just as each country has its own language and culture, each type of pneumococcus bacterium has unique traits. Some types tend to be more aggressive, while other types are more resistant to treatment. Neither the polysaccharide vaccine nor the conjugate vaccine protects you from all the types of pneumococcus, but these vaccines are designed to prevent infections from the most aggressive types.

Symptoms of Pneumococcal Infection

Symptoms can include:

- Fever
- Irritability

- Shortness of breath or rapid breathing
- Pain in the chest
- Chills
- Coughing

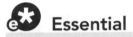 **Essential**

Even though pneumococcal infections are far more common than Hib infections, the pneumococcus bacterium is not as aggressive as the Hib bacterium. Generally, pneumococcus infections lead to fewer deaths, and the infections are more treatable with antibiotics.

Even though the pneumococcus bacterium causes the majority of bacterial pneumonia in young children, it is not the only infection that this bacterium causes. In addition, this bacterium is responsible for the vast majority of ear infections and blood infection in children.

How Does One Catch It?

The pneumococcus bacterium travels from one person to the next through the air. When a sick person coughs or sneezes, he sprays the bacteria into the air. An unsuspecting person nearby may breathe in the bacteria and get sick.

 Alert

What is so sneaky about this bacterium is that it can live in people's noses without making them sick. Just because the people around you do not appear sick does not mean that you will not get sick from them. Many people harbor this bacterium in their nose without realizing it.

While the pneumococcus bacterium is not as contagious as chickenpox or measles, it can still be passed quite readily through coughing and sneezing. Patients with pneumococcal infections should be quarantined to prevent an outbreak. Other than isolating yourself completely from any human contact, there is no effective way to always avoid getting exposed to the pneumococcus bacterium.

How Common Is the Infection?

Pneumococcal infections rank among the most common bacterial infections in the world. It is the most common cause of bacterial ear infection and pneumonia in children. It causes more blood infection in babies than any other bacterium.

 Fact

Before the pneumococcal conjugate vaccine was introduced, annually the pneumococcus bacterium caused 700 children to come down with brain infection, 17,000 children to have infection of their blood, and 71,000 children to develop pneumonia.

Each year, about 200 children less than five years old die from pneumococcal infections in the United States. In developing countries, this number is far higher.

How Serious Is the Infection?

Even though pneumococcus is not as dangerous as the Hib bacterium, it is still responsible for many life-threatening infections, such as bloodstream infection, pneumonia, brain infection, and sinus infection.

For people with reduced immune systems, this bacterium is even more dangerous. People suffering from the flu are especially susceptible to getting an infection from pneumococcus. When the immune system is not functioning optimally—such as with patients suffering from asthma or chronic liver disease, or patients undergoing chemotherapy—the chance of dying from this infection is a lot higher. In addition, babies younger than six months are more likely to have a brain infection than older children due to their immature immune system.

🅔❗ Alert

If your child's spleen has been damaged or surgically removed, she is more likely to suffer from serious pneumococcal infections than other children. The spleen's normal function is to filter out dangerous bacteria from the bloodstream. Ask your pediatrician whether your child needs additional protection from this bacterium if you are not sure.

Is the Infection Treatable?

Pneumococcal infections used to be readily treatable by antibiotics, but this is no longer the case. While some types of pneumococcus remains easy to treat, many types of pneumococcus bacterium have developed resistance to antibiotics. Stronger antibiotics must be used to treat these tough infections. It is not unforeseeable that sooner or later some strains of this bacterium will develop resistance to all antibiotics, rendering all treatment futile.

Since the pneumococcal vaccine became available, the pneumococcus bacterium has become less resistant to antibiotic treatment because the vaccine is targeted against those types of bacteria that are most likely to develop resistance to treatment.

Components of the Pneumococcal Vaccine

As mentioned previously, there are two types of pneumococcal vaccines. The polysaccharide pneumococcal vaccine is made from the outer covering of twenty-three types of the pneumococcus bacterium. There are a total of ninety different types of pneumococcus bacterium, so even the polysaccharide vaccine covers only a fraction of the total number of pneumococcal infections. However, the twenty-three types of bacterium are responsible for causing 85 to 90 percent of the most dangerous types of infection from pneumococcus. Even though the polysaccharide vaccine does not cover all the different types of pneumococcus bacterium, it still protects its recipient from more than 85 percent of serious pneumococcal infections.

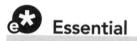 **Essential**

The pneumococcal polysaccharide or conjugate vaccines do not contain any preservatives, including thimerosal. In fact, there is no longer any mercury preservative in any of the vaccines given to children less than eleven years of age.

The pneumococcal conjugate vaccine protects against even less types of pneumococci bacteria. It only contains the covering chemical from seven types of pneumococcus bacterium. However, these seven types included in the conjugate vaccine are not selected randomly. The seven types of bacterium cause the majority (about 80 percent) of brain and blood infections in children. So even though the vaccine is designed to fight against so few types of the pneumococcus, it actually works quite well for the majority of the serious childhood pneumococcal infections.

In addition to the sugar coating on the pneumococcus bacterium, the conjugate vaccine also contains a protein from the diphtheria bacterium. This protein is a defective form of the diphtheria toxin, which is incapable of causing harm because of its defect. Similar to the Hib conjugate vaccine, this protein is connected to the pneumococcal conjugate vaccine to allow the immune system to recognize the sugar covering of the pneumococcus bacterium. Again, it is like shining a spotlight on the mug shot of the germ so the body will pay extra attention to this germ's profile.

A very small amount of aluminum is also present in the pneumococcal conjugate vaccine. This is similar to many other vaccines, including the Hib vaccine and the DTaP vaccine. The aluminum further draws attention of the immune system to the germ's chemicals when the injection is given. If you are concerned about the safety of aluminum in vaccines, please refer to Chapter 4 on vaccine safety.

Side Effects of the Pneumococcal Vaccine

The pneumococcal conjugate vaccine is quite safe. Nevertheless, it frequently causes mild reactions at the site of injection. Redness and mild swelling at the injection site are quite common, but they are short lasting. The skin reaction is rarely severe enough to prevent your child from playing and acting normally. In addition to these local reactions, your child may be more irritable or sleepy for one to two days after receiving the pneumococcal conjugate vaccine.

The pneumococcal vaccine has not been implicated with autoimmune disorders or autism. This vaccine never contained the mercury-based thimerosal or any other types of preservatives. Millions of doses of pneumococcal conjugate vaccine have been given, and the experience so far shows that no permanent side effects have been reported.

Fact

Beyond mild skin irritation at the injection site and a slight fever, there are no reported serious side effects that have been linked to the pneumococcal conjugate vaccine. This vaccine is not blamed for autism because the autism epidemic was already rampant by the time this vaccine was licensed.

Similar to most other vaccines, the pneumococcal vaccine can cause a fever. The chance of a high fever (temperature greater than 102°F) is about 2 percent, which is slightly higher than the chance of a high temperature after receiving the DTaP vaccine. This fever rarely lasts for more than three days, and the fever itself does not cause any harm to your child.

CHAPTER 12

The Rotavirus Vaccine

D espite being the most common cause of diarrhea in babies, rotavirus remains a relatively obscure bug for the general public. Chances are that you have never heard of this virus, yet this bug has been causing problem for hundreds of years. In 2006, a new vaccine against this virus became available, and it has already made a big impact in reducing hospitalization. However, a serious side effect tainted an older rotavirus vaccine, which was the reason the older version of this vaccine was taken off the market in 1999.

Introduction

There are two main reasons why scientists try to come up with a vaccine for an infection: either the infection is very serious or the infection is very common (and sometimes both situations are true). In the case of the rotavirus vaccine, it is because of the latter. Rotavirus infection is rarely life threatening in the United States, even though it is responsible for the deaths of half a million children around the world each year. The majority of deaths occur in developing countries where there is not easy access to a medical facility. In 2007, less than fifty American babies died from rotavirus infection.

The rotavirus vaccine works well to keep children out of the hospital. Even if the vaccine does not completely prevent diarrhea caused by this virus, it prevents hospital admission 96 percent of the time. The vaccine first became widely used in 2006, and the 2007–2008 rotavirus season was drastically different from previous years. Not only did the season arrive later, but the magnitude of the outbreak was significantly reduced.

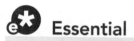 **Essential**

Your child does not become immune to this virus after a previous infection. However, the infection is usually less severe the second or third time around. Rotavirus does not pose a serious problem to older children and adults because they were probably exposed to this virus before.

The rotavirus vaccine differs from many other vaccines in that it is not injected into the body with a needle. Instead, this vaccine comes in a small single-dose vial and is administered directly into the mouth of your child from the prepackaged vial. The vaccine contains a very small amount of liquid (2 ml, or 2 cc, to be exact), and the direct administration of the vaccine without using a syringe avoids contamination of the vaccine.

 Fact

A new rotavirus vaccine became available in June 2008. It is called Rotarix, and it is similar to the RotaTeq vaccine. The difference between these two vaccines is that the virus in the Rotarix vaccine is weakened by a different method than the RotaTeq vaccine. Both vaccines have been demonstrated to be safe.

Three doses of the vaccine are routinely recommended—one at the two-month, one at the four-month, and one at the six-month visit. However, all three doses of this vaccine must be given within a small window of time. Unlike many other vaccines, where a catch-up dose can be given months or even years after the initial dose, the first dose of the rotavirus vaccine must be given prior to twelve weeks after birth, and the rotavirus vaccine cannot be given after thirty-two weeks of age (around eight months old). If your child missed this vaccine at the two-month well baby visit, she cannot get this vaccine at the four-month visit. The reason for this small window of time is that this vaccine has not been tested in younger infants and older infants. Whether this vaccine is safe for older children (children older than eight months) is unknown.

Alert

If your baby spits up some of the rotavirus vaccine right after it was administered, a repeat dose is not recommended. However, your baby can still get the remaining doses in the vaccine series.

Similar to the measles and chickenpox vaccine, the rotavirus vaccine contains live but weakened virus, so it should not be given to babies who have a defective immune system (such as infants with leukemia, lymphoma, or AIDS, or infants undergoing chemotherapy). If your baby had received a blood transfusion in the past six weeks, she should not receive the rotavirus vaccine until later.

Rotavirus Infection

Rotavirus causes severe diarrhea and vomiting in young children. The diarrhea can be quite relentless (more than twenty watery stools in a day), and it frequently lasts more than a week. Many children become dehydrated from this infection each year, but babies are especially vulnerable. The bodies of infants are small to begin with, and there is not as much water content in the small body compared to older children. Faced with a constant and massive stool loss, their small bodies can become dehydrated in a matter of hours.

As stated earlier, rotavirus infections are almost never fatal in the United States. The effects of dehydration can be reversed quickly with intravenous fluid, and the ready access to hospital care in this country makes death highly unlikely for a typical rotavirus infection. Nevertheless, tens of thousands of babies become hospitalized from this infection each year in the United States, and the duration of each hospitalization can last from just a few days to more than a week. Generally, the frequency of diarrhea must decrease to a reasonable level before the baby is discharged from the hospital.

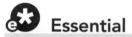 **Essential**

Diarrhea caused by rotavirus never contains blood. If your child experiences bloody diarrhea, she may be infected with a bacteria. See your doctor without delay if you find substances that resemble blood in your child's stool.

Symptoms of the Rotavirus Infection

Symptoms of a rotavirus infection include:

- Fever
- Vomiting
- Watery diarrhea (frequent)
- Abdominal pain
- Loss of interest in food

 Fact

Due to the frequency and severity of diarrhea, rotavirus infection can cause dehydration but also an imbalance of salts in the body. For this reason, daily blood tests are sometimes necessary to monitor the salt levels in the body. Serious imbalance of salts in the body can cause swelling of the brain, seizure, and even death.

How Does One Catch It?

Rotavirus infection is highly contagious, and it is transmitted mainly by contact with fecal-contaminated objects. Children are most vulnerable because their hygiene practice tends to be poor and many of them like to put things in their mouths. Adults, however, are not immune to this infection. Parents are especially prone to catching the infection from their children during diaper changes or cleaning up vomit.

A child with rotavirus infection can shed virus in the stool for up to three weeks. During this entire time, the stool remains contagious, and anyone who has direct contact with the child is susceptible to catching the infection.

Hand washing is the most effective way to avoid getting rotavirus infection. However, not all hand washers are created equal. Hand-washing duration and technique do matter, and a thorough cleaning offers more protection than a hasty attempt.

How Common Is the Infection?

Rotavirus is responsible for causing the majority of infectious diarrhea in children. Virtually all children have been infected by this virus by age five years. Each year in the United States, rotavirus causes 200,000 emergency room visits and more than 50,000 hospitalizations in children. Nevertheless, deaths from rotavirus infection are extremely rare in the United States.

The low rate of death is mainly attributable to the availability of emergency medical services in this country. The dehydration caused by rotavirus is easily reversible, so as long as caregivers bring their children to a medical facility in a timely manner, serious problems resulting from diarrhea is almost always averted.

On the other hand, this vaccine can potentially save millions of lives around the world. Medical care is a luxury in many parts of the world, and more than half a million babies die from rotavirus infection each year. A global immunization effort is under way to distribute this vaccine so it can be widely available in developing countries.

How Serious Is the Infection?

Rotavirus infection is rarely deadly in the United States. Dehydration that results from the nonstop vomiting and diarrhea can be readily reversed by using intravenous fluid. As long as parents bring their sick children to the hospital promptly, babies almost never die from this infection.

An imbalance of salt levels and a buildup of acid can also result from the severe dehydration triggered by rotavirus infection. Doctors routinely monitor the concentration of salts and acid in babies who have severe diarrhea secondary to rotavirus infection. Fortunately, these complications are readily reversible if detected, and permanent disability from salt imbalance is extremely rare.

Despite its relatively benign course, the rotavirus infection is estimated to be responsible for about half a million doctor's visit each year. Of all those who are evaluated, more than 50,000 children end up in the hospital because of moderate to severe dehydration.

Is the Infection Treatable?

The rotavirus is a virus, so antibiotics are useless against this infection. Medications used by adults to slow down diarrhea can be dangerous when used in children, so you should never give your baby over-the-counter antidiarrheal medications (such as Immodium).

The only treatment available during a rotavirus infection is offering your child plenty of liquid to drink. If your baby has a lot of vomiting and cannot keep down any fluid, he would most likely need to be hospitalized and receive intravenous therapy.

Hospitalization for dehydration caused by rotavirus is usually short—two to three days. After your baby leaves the hospital, no long-term treatment would be necessary. Occasionally, if the vomiting and diarrhea were severe, a follow-up appointment with the doctor would be necessary after discharge to ensure that your baby is able to keep drinking and avoid dehydration.

Components of the Rotavirus Vaccine

The rotavirus vaccine contains live rotavirus that has been genetically altered so it is no longer harmful. However, these vaccine viruses retain enough characteristics of the wild rotavirus to alert the immune system so that when the regular rotavirus comes along your child's body knows exactly how to handle this germ.

In addition to the rotavirus, this vaccine also has a trace amount of blood cells from cows. The vaccine virus was grown in cow's blood, so when the virus was extracted from its growth liquid, a small amount of cow's blood also gets into the vaccine. This small amount of blood could trigger an allergic reaction in extremely rare circumstances in some people.

 Fact

The rotavirus vaccine does not and never did contain the mercury-based preservative thimerosal. In fact, this vaccine contains no preservative whatsoever. Since this vaccine contains live virus, thimerosal would render the vaccine useless because any preservative would kill the live virus.

Finally, the rotavirus vaccine also contains a small amount of salt and sugar. These components do not cause any allergic reaction or harmful side effects.

Side Effects of the Rotavirus Vaccine

In 1998, the pharmaceutical company Wyeth introduced the first vaccine against rotavirus to the market. The vaccine was called RotaShield, and it worked well. But just as the number of children stricken by this virus was trending down, some doctors became alarmed because a few babies suffered intestinal obstruction following this vaccination. The Centers for Disease Control and Prevention (CDC) looked into this matter and found that there is a small but definite risk for intussusception after the old rotavirus vaccine was given. Less than a year after this vaccine became available, the RotaShield vaccine was pulled off the market.

Intussusception is a blockage of the intestines. It occurs when one segment of the intestine becomes trapped in an adjacent segment, similar to successive segments of a collapsible antenna or telescope. This condition is a medical emergency. Unless the blockage is reversed, the intestine could become swollen and bacteria could leak out from inside the intestine to the entire body. Intussusception can be treated with an enema or with surgery. The treatment must be instituted quickly with either modality before the condition worsens. Even though surgery for intussusception carries a slightly higher risk, surgery tends to fix the problem most of the time. Occasionally the enema would temporarily fix the blockage, but the intussusception can return at a later time. If an enema fails to resolve the blockage, surgery would be necessary to make this problem go away. Fifteen percent of babies with intussusception die from the condition, mostly because of a delay in diagnosis.

The symptoms of intussusception include drowsiness, abdominal cramps, bloody stools, vomiting, and loss of consciousness. If diagnosed early, the problem is easily reversible. However, intussusception can be very difficult to recognize early in the course of the disease. Often the condition is misdiagnosed as stomach flu, and the delay in treatment can be disastrous. If left untreated, intussusception is almost always fatal.

The old RotaShield rotavirus vaccine was not the only cause of intussusception. In fact, the vast majority of intussusception occurs spontaneously, which means that scientists are not sure why this rare condition occurs in some babies. Intussusception occurs most commonly after a stomach infection, and there is some evidence that shows the new rotavirus vaccine can actually prevent some cases of intussusception. This finding has not been confirmed, so you should not think the main role of the rotavirus vaccine is to prevent intussusception.

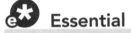 **Essential**

The risk for intussusception after the RotaShield vaccine was approximately 1 in 10,000 doses. This complication is rare, but not rare enough to accept the risk. The new RotaTeq vaccine was introduced in 2006, and intussusception has not occurred resulting from the administration of this new vaccine.

When the new rotavirus vaccine, RotaTeq, was invented, the potential risk of intussusception was on the mind of all the scientists working on the vaccine. It would be pointless to introduce another rotavirus vaccine if the new vaccine could also cause intussusception. The possibility of intussusception was thoroughly studied during the clinical trial of the new RotaTeq vaccine, and an unprecedentedly large clinical research was conducted to look for the chance of intussusception after the administration of the new RotaTeq vaccine. After thoroughly analyzing the data, scientists conclude that there is no increased risk for intussusception after receiving the new rotavirus vaccine.

Beside intussusception, there is an additional concern about this vaccine. Because the rotavirus vaccine contains live virus, babies who received this vaccine shed the vaccine virus afterward. There is a theoretical risk for this vaccine virus to be passed on to susceptible individuals. This is the reason why individuals in the same household whose immune system is weakened should stay away from babies who just had the rotavirus vaccine.

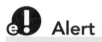 **Alert**

Having household members with weakened immune systems is not a reason to postpone administering the rotavirus vaccine. The chance of spreading the weakened rotavirus in the vaccine to another household member is extremely small, and the benefit of the vaccine for the baby outweighs the risk of possible exposure to the vaccine virus.

There have been some concerns that the rotavirus vaccine may be linked to a condition called Kawasaki disease. Kawasaki disease is a rare condition where blood vessels in the body become irritated. However, since this concern was raised, there have been numerous studies that have refuted any connection between the new rotavirus vaccine and Kawasaki disease. Most experts agree that the rotavirus vaccine does not trigger Kawasaki disease.

CHAPTER 13

The MMR Vaccine

The MMR vaccine is infamous for its association with autism. Many parents believe that the MMR vaccine is primarily responsible for the recent global epidemic of autism. On the other hand, there is strong evidence that shows autism continues to increase in communities despite complete cessation of the use of the MMR vaccine. Nevertheless, the controversy continues because the scourge of autism remains rampant and emotions run high in a time of crisis.

Introduction

The MMR vaccine is a combination vaccine that contains components that protect against three different germs—measles, mumps, and rubella. The MMR vaccine has not always been a combination vaccine. At one point, the vaccines for measles, mumps, and rubella were three separate vaccines. These three individual vaccines were all invented in the same decade—measles vaccine in 1963, mumps vaccine in 1967, and the rubella vaccine in 1969. Since all three vaccines were made from live viruses, it was not difficult to combine them into one shot to reduce the number of injections children get. In 1971, the MMR combination vaccine was introduced in the United States by the Merck pharmaceutical company. Merck still manufactures the vast majority of the MMR vaccine used in the United States today.

Essential

It used to be possible to obtain individual vaccines for measles, mumps, and rubella. However, the vaccine manufacturing companies ceased production of these individual vaccines in 2009, making them extremely hard to come by.

When the MMR vaccine first became available, doctors only recommended one dose of the MMR vaccine at age twelve months, but this vaccine regimen only protected 95 percent of all children from these infections. Even though 95 percent may sound really good to you, it was not good enough to prevent some children from dying of measles. The American Academy of Pediatrics decided in 1989 to recommend a second booster shot for the MMR vaccine at age four year, which is right before many children first enter school. This second dose of vaccine boosts the effectiveness of the vaccine to more than 99 percent.

Fact

The MMR vaccine is sometimes combined with the chickenpox vaccine. This combination, also known as the MMRV vaccine (the V is for *varicella*, the medical term for chickenpox), first became available in 2005. There has been intermittent shortages of the MMRV combination vaccine, so your doctor may not have this new combination vaccine available.

The MMR vaccine can be administered at the same time as other vaccines. However, if another vaccine containing live virus is not given at the same time as the MMR vaccine, the other live-virus vaccine (frequently the chickenpox vaccine) must be postponed for at least twenty-eight days after the MMR vaccine. If two vaccines containing live virus are given too close together, they may interfere with each other and can cancel out each other's effect.

Ever since the introduction of the second MMR vaccine booster, measles infection has become relatively rare in America. Most parents have never seen a child with measles, due to the drastic reduction in the chance of catching this highly contagious infection.

Many adults have never had measles or received the measles vaccine. If you were born after 1956 and have never had the measles vaccine, you should talk to your doctor to see whether you should get vaccinated against measles. If you do not remember whether you had the measles vaccine or cannot find any record of your immunization, there is a blood test that can be done to find out whether you have been exposed to measles. If there is no evidence of immunity against measles, you should seriously consider getting the measles vaccine to protect yourself.

Most people mistakenly believe that they have had the measles infection in the past when in fact they have not. Many other viral infections can mimic the measles infection. So simply having a recollection of a measles infection does not prove that one is immune to measles. Immunity can only be proven with an immunization documentation in the medical record or with a blood test.

Adults who are returning to school to get their college degree may be required to show proof of immunity against measles. You can either provide a copy of your immunization record or you can have a blood test done to demonstrate that you have the antibody against the measles virus. If you have never had the vaccine or the infection, you would need two doses of the MMR vaccine, administered at least four weeks apart.

Measles

Measles is literally your parents' infection. The vaccine for measles first became available in the early 1960s, so most of you reading this book have been vaccinated and have never known a child with measles. However, there have been several outbreaks of measles in the United States in the past twenty years, because this infection is extremely contagious and a single dose of this vaccine only protects children from measles 95 percent of the time. This means that up to 5 percent of the individuals in school could still get measles despite timely vaccination. For something as contagious as measles, 5 percent of the population is enough to trigger a massive outbreak in a community.

😲 Alert

The most recent measles outbreak in the United States occurred in May 2008. Fourteen people were hospitalized during the outbreak, but fortunately no one died. The majority of those infected during the outbreak were not fully vaccinated against measles.

In the early 1990s, most school children had not received two doses of the measles vaccine. A major outbreak in the United States claimed the lives of 120 people and hospitalized more than 10,000. This tells you the vulnerability of the population to an infectious outbreak even when a vaccine works 95 percent of the time. More recent measles outbreaks were attributed to the reduction of immunization in school-aged children. Today, up to half of the children in schools are not vaccinated against measles in some communities due to concern regarding the relationship between the MMR vaccine and autism.

Currently, a large percentage of children in Great Britain have not received the MMR vaccine due to parents' fear of autism. Shortly following the drop in vaccination rate, measles outbreaks started almost immediately in many parts of the country. It is yet to be seen whether a large-scale epidemic of measles will spread through all of Europe in the near future.

Symptoms of the Measles Infection

Symptoms of the measles infection include:

- Fever
- Fatigue
- Dry cough
- Runny nose
- Bloodshot eyes
- Sore throat
- Headache
- Sensitivity to light
- Tiny white spots found inside the mouth
- Rash of large, red, flat blotches that often merge
- Can lead to inflammation and swelling of the brain

Measles in the United States today is very rare. Most recently trained pediatricians have never seen a child with measles, so it is not uncommon for the diagnosis to be delayed until much later.

✅ Fact

Prior to widespread childhood immunization, measles infection was so common that virtually everyone had been infected with measles by the time they were adolescents. In a close-knit community, measles can spread like wildfire in a population that is not immunized.

How Does One Catch It?

Measles is highly contagious. It can spread by direct contact with secretions or through the air. Commercial air travel facilitates the spread of this infection by forcing a large group of travelers to congregate in a confined space for a long period of time. If a person with measles coughs, sneezes, or just talks to you, you may be infected with measles.

If you are exposed to a confirmed case of measles, you can receive immunoglobulin (a type of antibody) to protect you from coming down with the infection. This treatment must be given expeditiously to be effective.

How Common Is the Infection?

Due to the high immunization rate in the last thirty years, measles is rare in the United States. In 2005, only sixty-six people got measles in the United States. Half of them got measles that year as a result of a seventeen-year-old American traveler returning from Romania. He never received the measles vaccine.

While measles is uncommon in developed countries, it is still rampant in the rest of the world. About 3 million people get sick from measles each year around the world. The ease of worldwide travel makes this infection a real threat for American children. Unvaccinated travelers and immigrants continue to bring this infection back to the United States. The number of children vaccinated against measles continues to drop, and it is just a matter of time before another measles outbreak spreads through your community.

🅔❗ Alert

Even though measles is rare in the United States, it is still a major threat to children in the rest of the world. Of all the infections that can be prevented by vaccination, measles kills more children around the world than any other infection. Each year, about one million children die from measles in the world.

Besides universal measles vaccination, the only way to prevent future measles outbreaks in the United States is to ban everyone from traveling in and out of this country. A complete nationwide quarantine would be necessary to stop travelers from bringing measles into the country.

How Serious Is the Infection?

Measles can lead to permanent brain damage. About 1 out of 1,000 children with measles will develop swelling of the brain, and 10 to 15 percent of them will die from the infection.

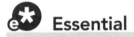 **Essential**

Babies younger than a year of age are too young to receive the measles vaccination. They rely on older children around them being immune to the infection so they will not get sick from measles. Young infants also derive some protection from the antibody they receive from their mothers during pregnancy.

The vast majority of the time, however, measles is not a fatal illness. Nevertheless, it can cause pneumonia, ear infection, croup, and inflammation of the liver.

Is the Infection Treatable?

There is no effective treatment for measles. Doctors can administer medications to reduce the swelling in the brain and prescribe antibiotics for pneumonia and ear infection, but these treatments do not affect the measles infection itself.

Sometimes expensive immunoglobulin is given as a last-ditch effort to treat patients with life-threatening complications, but this therapy has not demonstrated any efficacy in past experience. If immunoglobulin is given to a child who was exposed to measles but has not actually gotten sick from it, it may help to prevent the infection.

Mumps

The image of a chipmunk may come to mind when you hear of mumps. This is because when children have mumps, their cheeks swell up to make them resemble these wild rodents. Though the image may be comical, mumps can sometimes cause serious complications, including the loss of reproductive function in males.

The swelling of the face with mumps infection is caused by inflammation of the glands in the cheeks that make saliva. Most people who come down with mumps end up with swelling, but this problem fortunately does not cause any serious long-term issues.

Before the mumps vaccine was combined with the measles and rubella vaccine, it was a stand-alone vaccine. There is an interesting back story about the invention of the mumps vaccine. In fact, the inventor of the mumps vaccine is an even more interesting character. The man behind the vaccine was Maurice Hilleman.

Maurice Hilleman had a humble beginning. He was raised in rural Montana, and his mother died when she was giving birth to his twin sisters. He was brought up to be self-reliant and he grew up to be a practical man. He never allowed politics or business to get in the way of saving lives.

Maurice Hilleman's unparalleled achievement in the development of childhood vaccines ranks him among the greatest scientists—with Louis Pasteur and Edward Jenner. However, most people have probably never heard of this guy because he contributed to science quietly. He never won the Nobel Prize because he did not work in academia. Instead, he was involved in inventing more than a half dozen childhood vaccines that are currently used today, including vaccines against measles, mumps, rubella, chickenpox, bacterial meningitis, flu, and hepatitis B.

In 1957, while reading a newspaper report about a flu outbreak in Hong Kong, he took a look at a photograph of a group of sick children, and he immediately realized that a flu pandemic was on the way to the United States. He promptly started a race to come up with the first pandemic flu vaccine. After working fourteen hours a day and inoculating 150,000 chicken eggs himself, the United States had the first pandemic flu vaccine. An estimated one million Americans were expected to die from the pandemic flu that year. Forty million doses of the pandemic flu vaccine were eventually given, and the death toll was reduced to 69,000 from that year's flu outbreak. Most people credit Maurice Hilleman for saving tens of thousands of American lives.

On an early morning in March 1963, Maurice was scheduled to travel to South America, but his five-year-old daughter, Jeryl Lynn, woke him up from his sleep. She had a high fever. Being an astute practical scientist, Maurice immediately recognized that his daughter had mumps. So he comforted her like any good father would, but then he did something that no ordinary father does. In the middle of the night, he drove in to his laboratory at work and took a cotton swab. He came back home and got a sample from Jeryl Lynn's throat, and he went back to the laboratory and transferred the mumps virus from his daughter's throat into a culture broth. Later that morning, he flew to South America for his business trip. When he returned, he found out that he had indeed isolated the mumps virus from his daughter, and using that virus, he came up with the first working mumps vaccine. This is still the same mumps vaccine that is being used today, and the virus in the vaccine is called the Jeryl Lynn strain, named after his daughter.

Symptoms of the Mumps Infection

Symptoms of the mumps infection include:

- Fever
- Headache
- Muscle aches
- Fatigue
- Loss of appetite
- Swollen salivary glands

How Does One Catch It?

Mumps is passed on by direct transfer of the salivary secretion. Sharing utensils or a cup with an infected person is a common way to catch this infection. In rare circumstances, it can be transmitted by air when an affected person coughs or sneezes. While mumps is not as contagious as measles, outbreaks can still occur in communities where people are not fully vaccinated.

How Common Is the Infection?

Mumps has become a very rare infection since vaccination against it started in 1967. However, it has been observed that outbreaks can still occur in population where up to 96 percent of the people are vaccinated against it. In 2003, less than 500 cases of mumps were reported.

How Serious Is the Infection?

Mumps is generally a very mild infection, especially in children. Rare complications can affect older adults, including painful swelling of the testicles that can lead to sterility and deafness. The vast majority of children with mumps recover from the swelling of the salivary glands without any long-term complications.

🔔 Alert

In extremely rare circumstances, mumps can cause breast inflammation, meningitis, and even miscarriages. However, birth defects from infection during pregnancy have never been observed.

Meningitis, or infection of the covering surrounding the brain, can occur with mumps infection about 10 percent of the time. A spinal tap is necessary to make this diagnosis. Fortunately, children with mumps meningitis usually recover completely, but hospitalization for two to three days may be necessary.

Encephalitis, or infection of the brain, can be caused by mumps very rarely (about 2 in 100,000 cases of mumps). About 1 percent of children afflicted with mumps encephalitis will die.

Is the Infection Treatable?

There is no known treatment for mumps. Drinking plenty of fluid and resting are recommended if your child comes down with mumps. Fever reducers and pain relievers can be used to ameliorate the symptoms of mumps. The rare complications from mumps cannot be treated or prevented.

Rubella

The MMR vaccine should really be known as the autism vaccine. It earns this reputation not because the vaccine triggers autism, but it can prevent autism. More specifically, the rubella component of the vaccine can prevent congenital rubella syndrome in babies. Autism, or profound mental retardation, is the primary and most devastating complication of congenital rubella syndrome.

 Fact

As a side effect of the rubella scourge of the 1960s, the abortion rate spiked because desperate mothers attempted to terminate their pregnancies to avoid giving birth to severely deformed and retarded babies.

Rubella (German measles) does not cause a serious illness for children and adults. At most, a mild fever with a rash and some joint pain is all that there is to it when the infection strikes. But if a pregnant woman gets the infection during the first three months of pregnancy, the fetus would most likely suffer birth defects. Similar to polio, rubella became a much more serious problem when sanitation and the standard of living improved in this country. Instead of getting the infection during infancy or childhood, girls managed to stay away from the infection until they became women. Suddenly in the 1960s, a large number of women were miscarrying or giving birth to babies who were blind, deaf, and retarded. Congenital rubella became a national scourge in the 1960s.

Between 1964 and 1965, rubella devastated the nation, leading to more than 10,000 miscarriages and more than 25,000 babies born with severe birth defects. Many of these children ended as wards of the state because social services were not available at the time to place children with special needs. Even devoted parents eventually gave up these children because the parents were unable to communicate with and care for them.

Symptoms of the Rubella Infection

Symptoms of a rubella infection include:

- Fever
- Headache
- Fatigue
- Runny nose
- Swollen or tender lymph nodes
- Bloodshot eyes
- Muscle or joint pain
- Rash with pink or red spots (rash may merge to form patches and can be itchy)

How Does One Catch It?

Rubella is easily transmitted from one person to another by contact or through the air. Most people catch the infection in late winter and early spring. Pregnant women often get exposed to rubella from unvaccinated school-age children, frequently from their own children.

When children get the infection, they often exhibit no symptoms at all. Since it is impossible to tell who might have rubella, this infection cannot be prevented by avoiding sick people. Rubella is most contagious when the rash associated with it is visible, but for many people, the rash never appears.

How Common Is the Infection?

In the early 1960s, rubella was rampant in the United States. More than 12 million people were diagnosed with rubella, and more than 20,000 babies were disabled by congenital rubella syndrome.

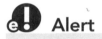 **Alert**

> Rubella can be devastating to a fetus if a pregnant woman contracts the disease. Many children become mentally retarded or have serious heart problems resulting from congenital rubella syndrome.

However, that statistic is just a history lesson. Congenital rubella syndrome is now extremely rare in the United States. In the past ten years, less than ten babies were born with congenital rubella syndrome. The massive epidemic of rubella is now a distant memory.

How Serious Is the Infection?

The rubella infection itself does not cause any serious problems. If rubella strikes a child or a grown man, it is an inconsequential illness. It only causes problems when a pregnant woman catches the infection.

Babies with congenital rubella syndrome are almost always born very small, and eight out of ten babies born to mothers who were infected with rubella are deformed or disabled. Deafness is the most common permanent problem associated with congenital rubella syndrome. About 60 percent of children with congenital rubella syndrome are severely hearing impaired. Approximately 40 percent of these children are born with cataract, glaucoma, and retinal abnormalities. Heart problems affect many of these children as well, and sometimes heart problems can be fatal if diagnosis is delayed.

Behavioral problems that are similar or indistinguishable from autism commonly affect children with congenital rubella syndrome, and many children are mentally retarded. Congenital rubella syndrome is one of the few known causes of autism.

⊛ Essential

Congenital rubella syndrome is most likely to occur if the pregnant woman gets infected during the first trimester of the pregnancy. If she gets sick after the second trimester, congenital rubella syndrome virtually never occurs.

Is the Infection Treatable?

The rubella infection itself does not require treatment because it is a mild illness that gets better on its own. Congenital rubella syndrome, on the other hand, cannot be treated because the damage to the baby has already been done to the fetus by the time the baby is born.

Various corrective measures are available to fix the birth defects. Eye surgery can replace the diseased lenses in the eyes, and hearing aids are available to partially restore hearing in some individuals. The brain damage that occurs in some people is irreversible. Special adaptive lesson plans in school may help these children to learn and become more independent, but they will never function at the same level as their healthy peers.

Components of the MMR Vaccine

The MMR vaccine contains live viruses grown in the laboratory. These viruses differ from the regular measles, mumps, and rubella virus because they have been weakened by growing in an unfriendly environment. While these viruses in the MMR vaccine remain alive, they are incapable of causing the infection itself.

In addition to the weakened viruses, the MMR vaccine also contains a miniscule amount of egg protein because the viruses were grown in the laboratory using chicken cells.

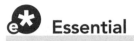 **Essential**

The MMR vaccine does not contain any preservatives or adjuvant. Preservatives and adjuvant (most commonly aluminum) cannot be used in vaccines containing live viruses because these chemicals would inactivate the vaccine and render it useless. The MMR vaccine never contained any thimerosal preservative.

A small amount of sugar is present in the MMR vaccine. Human protein and a trace of the antibiotic neomycin are also present in the vaccine. The antibiotic is necessary to prevent bacterial contamination of the vaccine during storage and transport.

Side Effects of the MMR Vaccine

Most children experience no reaction after receiving the MMR vaccine, but about 15 percent of them can have a fever a week after the vaccination. The fever is usually mild, but it can be as high as 103°F. Even though high temperature can be worrisome for a parent, the fever generally goes away on its own in one to two days. About 5 percent of children may develop a rash seven to ten days after the immunization. The rash is not itchy, and it also goes away in a few days without treatment.

However, parents are not generally too concerned about these relatively minor and transient reactions after the MMR vaccine. The main concern with the MMR vaccine is the possible link between the MMR vaccine and autism.

Autism inevitably gets diagnosed after the MMR vaccine was given. One of the central characteristics of autistic children is their inability to communicate effectively. Most autistic children cannot carry on a conversation easily.

At the same time, healthy children before their first birthdays cannot communicate effectively anyway. Due to this inability to evaluate speech, diagnosing autism before the age of one is quite difficult, but it is not impossible. Since the first dose of the MMR vaccine is administered after one year of age, autism is almost always diagnosed after the first dose of the MMR vaccine.

✅ Fact

More than 90 percent of autism is diagnosed after twelve months of age. Only highly trained child development specialists have enough experience to diagnose autistic children before their first birthday, and even their diagnoses are not correct all the time at this young age.

This is the reason why parents of autistic children say that their children became autistic after the MMR vaccine. It is challenging to diagnose autism prior to the age of one year. For an in-depth discussion of autism and vaccination, please refer to Chapter 5 of this book.

Since the virus in the MMR vaccine is cultured in young chicken cells, many parents are concerned that if their child is allergic to chicken egg, there is the possibility of an allergic reaction after getting the MMR vaccine. Rigorous analysis of this possibility has demonstrated that individuals with egg allergy do not experience any allergic reaction after getting the MMR vaccine. However, this is not the case for the flu vaccine. Individuals with severe egg allergy should not receive the flu vaccine because the flu vaccine contains significantly higher concentration of egg protein than the MMR vaccine.

Separating the MMR Vaccine

Even though there is very strong evidence that shows the MMR vaccine does not cause autism, some parents are still worried and want to obtain the MMR vaccine in separated vaccines. Following are specific instructions on how to procure the individual vaccines for your child.

 Alert

> The vaccine manufacturing companies ceased production of the individual MMR vaccines in early 2009, making these individual vaccines extremely hard to come by. Most medical offices do not carry these individual vaccines anymore.

First, make sure your doctor agrees to order and administering the separated vaccines. Most doctors do not recommend separating the shots and may not accommodate your request.

After you find a doctor who is supportive, ask her to write a prescription for the following individual vaccines:

- **Attenuvax** (the measles vaccine)
- **Mumpsvax** (the mumps vaccine)
- **Meruvax** (the rubella vaccine)

All three vaccines are manufactured by the Merck pharmaceutical company. Get the address and telephone number to your doctor's office, and call the vaccine distributor American Medicine at (225)924-0247. Provide the distributor with your doctor's contact and shipping information, and fax your doctor's prescription to (225)924-0249. You will also need to provide your billing information. Health insurance companies generally do not reimburse for these individual vaccines.

✱ Essential

If you have the vaccines shipped to your own address, keep the vaccines refrigerated until the doctor is ready to administer them. In addition, keep the vaccines out of direct sunlight, because sunlight may inactivate these vaccines.

Vaccine manufacturers typically do not sell a single dose of these individual vaccines, so you may need to order a ten-dose pack of these vaccines. The vaccine distributor will ship the vaccines to your doctor's office via overnight shipping. The total cost of the vaccines plus shipping is about $150. Many parents donate the remaining vaccines to the doctor's office or to other parents who wish to get the separated vaccines.

CHAPTER 14

The Chickenpox Vaccine

S ome parents are surprised that there is a vaccine for chickenpox. Most parents have probably experienced chickenpox firsthand as a child and may wonder why it is necessary to vaccinate children when most people recover from chickenpox unscathed. Furthermore, the chickenpox vaccine contains live virus, and this adds more unease for some parents about subjecting their children to this vaccine. This chapter will discuss the rationale behind this vaccine and address concerns about its side effects.

Introduction

You may think that chickenpox is a harmless disease, so why bother having a vaccine for it? Chickenpox is relatively benign. The vast majority of children with chickenpox recover from it with just a few barely visible scars on the body. However, a small percentage of children may suffer serious complications from the chickenpox infection. Even though the chance of having a serious problem with chickenpox is so small, this group of people may add up to a sizable number since chickenpox is so common. Before the chickenpox vaccine became available, almost every single child got the chickenpox before reaching adulthood.

To prevent the 10,000 hospitalizations and few cases of death each year, the chickenpox vaccine was licensed in 1995. Initially, only a single dose of this vaccine was recommended for children twelve months or older. However, the chickenpox vaccine was only 85 percent effective in preventing chickenpox if only one dose was given. Currently two doses of the chickenpox vaccine are recommended. The first dose is usually given at the one-year visit, and the second dose is routinely scheduled at the four-year visit. Adolescents who only had a single dose when they were younger can get the booster dose at any time as long as it has been more than four weeks after their first chickenpox shot.

Alert

Since adults who catch chickenpox typically have a more severe case of the disease, adults are recommended to get two doses of the chickenpox vaccine. The two doses should be separated by at least four weeks for optimal efficacy.

Aside from some people questioning the necessity of the vaccine, another aspect of the chickenpox vaccine that makes it more controversial is that contains live chickenpox virus. When your child receives the vaccine, she in effect gets a very mild case of chickenpox. For most children, the symptoms are so mild that they are not even noticeable. About 5 percent of children who receive the chickenpox vaccine can have a fever and rash after vaccination. However, this mild form of chickenpox never causes complications such as pneumonia or death. Usually the rash is so mild that it may be confused with bug bites.

The chickenpox vaccine can be combined with the MMR vaccine as a four-in-one injection. The pharmaceutical company Merck has made this combination vaccine (often referred to as the MMRV vaccine) available since 2005. However, there was a nationwide shortage of this combination vaccine in 2008, and the shortage is ongoing at the time this book was published.

If the chickenpox vaccine is not given at the same time as the MMR vaccine, these two vaccines must be spaced at least twenty-eight days apart. Since both of these vaccines contain live viruses, they can interfere with each other if they are given too close together (unless they are given simultaneously).

 Question

If my child has already had chickenpox, does she still need to get the chickenpox vaccine?
If a doctor diagnosed your child with chickenpox in the past, it is not necessary to get the chickenpox vaccine. However, if your child received the chickenpox vaccine after a natural chickenpox infection, there is no harm done either.

Chickenpox Infection

Varicella is the medical term for chickenpox. The most common infection caused by the chickenpox virus is chickenpox, but the same virus can also cause shingles. Shingles is a painful sore on the face or body that erupts in mostly older individuals.

Fact

Ten to twenty percent of people who recover from chickenpox can develop shingles later in life. While most people experience shingles as older adults, shingles can flare up at any age, including during childhood.

The chickenpox virus is a close relative of the herpes virus that causes genital herpes in humans. Just like the herpes virus, the chickenpox virus incorporates its own DNA into your DNA and literally becomes a part of you after an infection. Even after your child recovers from the visible signs of chickenpox, the virus has already become part of your child, and it never leaves the body for the rest of your child's life. This is the reason why the chickenpox virus can remain dormant in the body for decades and reactivate later in life to manifest itself as shingles.

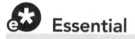 **Essential**

Even though pneumonia is a relatively uncommon complication of chickenpox, it is impossible to predict which child is going to come down with pneumonia with chickenpox. Some healthy children experience serious problems with chickenpox infection even though they have strong immune systems.

Chickenpox infection can be so mild in young children that it may not be recognized at the time of infection. Some adults who do not recall ever having chickenpox have an antibody against the virus. This means that these individuals probably had a very mild case of chickenpox when they were young, and the infection came and went unnoticed.

Symptoms of the Chickenpox Infection

Symptoms of a chickenpox infection include:

- Red, itchy rash (may initially look like bug bites or pimples)
- Small liquid-filled blisters that break and crust over
- Fever
- Mild headache
- Irritability
- Runny nose
- Sore throat
- Loss of appetite or abdominal pain
- Dry cough
- Pneumonia (rare)

How Does One Catch It?

The chickenpox virus spreads through the air and by direct contact. It is one of the most contagious germs known to man. If a person with chickenpox walks into a room, stays for a few minutes, leaves the room, and another person walks into the same room, the second person could get chickenpox. A whiff of air is all it takes to get sick from chickenpox.

 Fact

Unlike cowpox, which humans can get from cows, chickenpox has nothing to do with chickens. You cannot get chickenpox from chickens. The name "chickenpox" was derived from the appearance of the rash, which resembles chick peas.

What makes it even worse is that a person with chickenpox is already contagious a day or two before the rash appears. So a person may be spreading chickenpox without knowing it until it's too late. In addition, chickenpox remains contagious until all the blisters crust over, which can take more than two weeks for some people.

The incubation period for chickenpox is around two to three weeks. So if your child has been exposed to chickenpox, you will have to wait a few weeks before you know whether she will come down with chickenpox.

How Common Is the Infection?

Due to the highly contagious nature of this virus, chickenpox is extremely common. About 4 million children get chickenpox each year in the United States. More than 90 percent of adults have had the infection, and the most common age to get chickenpox is between the ages of four to ten in the United States. Chickenpox is relatively uncommon in babies.

Question

How do you know for sure whether you and your child have had chickenpox already?
There is a reliable blood test that checks for the presence of antibody against chickenpox in the body to confirm or refute a previous exposure to chickenpox. If the blood test confirms the presence of antibody against chickenpox in your child, your child does not need to get the chickenpox vaccine.

How Serious Is the Infection?

The vast majority of children with chickenpox recover completely without suffering any permanent disability. A few scars here and there are likely after recovering from chickenpox, but that is usually the extent of complication from the infection.

Fact

Chickenpox in pregnant women can cause birth defects, including blindness, brain damage, and permanent scarring of the skin or limbs for the fetus. The infection is especially dangerous during the first trimester of the pregnancy.

In rare circumstances, and especially in individuals with weakened immune systems (premature babies, people with AIDS), serious problems could result from chickenpox. Pneumonia is the most common complication, but brain infection (encephalitis) and life-threatening skin infection are also dangerous. Skin and soft tissue infection caused by chickenpox can often lead to amputation of the limbs. The difficult job of preventing these serious complications is that it is impossible to predict who may experience these life-threatening problems in advance. Many healthy children get extremely sick with chickenpox without having any risk factors. About a hundred people die from chickenpox infection each year in the United States.

Chickenpox is more serious if an adult catches it. Most babies who get chickenpox have rather mild symptoms. Adults account for more than half of the deaths from chickenpox.

Is the Infection Treatable?

No specific treatment is available for chickenpox, even though some antiviral medications have been shown to have modest effect against this virus. Most children just require topical lotion to alleviate the itching and fever reducer to provide comfort.

 Alert

You must never use aspirin in children with chickenpox. If children take aspirin when they have the chickenpox or the flu, they can experience a very dangerous reaction called Reye's syndrome. Reye's syndrome causes liver damage and permanent brain damage. Death can occur swiftly (in a matter of few hours) with Reye's syndrome.

While antibiotics are not effective against the chickenpox virus, they are often used to treat secondary bacterial infections that can complicate chickenpox, such as pneumonia and skin infections.

Components of the Chickenpox Vaccine

In addition to containing live but weakened chickenpox virus, the chickenpox vaccine also contains antibiotics to prevent bacterial contamination of the vaccine. The antibiotic used is neomycin, which is a common ingredient in topical antibiotics used for cuts and scrapes.

The vaccine contains gelatin, which could trigger an allergic reaction in rare circumstances. The chickenpox vaccine also contains sugar, salts, and trace amounts of the human lung cells used to grow the virus in laboratory. None of these components in the vaccine has ever caused any allergic reaction in humans.

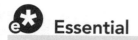 **Essential**

If your child is severely allergic to the antibiotic neomycin, she should not receive the chickenpox vaccine. If you are unsure, ask your doctor to have your child tested for possible allergy to this antibiotic prior to administering the chickenpox vaccine to your child.

Side Effects of the Chickenpox Vaccine

Since the chickenpox vaccine contains live but weakened chickenpox virus, the vaccine can trigger a mild case of chickenpox in about 5 percent of individuals after receiving the vaccine. A low-grade fever and rash usually does not develop until more than ten days after vaccination, and the symptoms are always mild. The rash that occurs after the vaccine usually has no more than thirty pimples throughout the body, compared to an average of 250 lesions in a typical case of chickenpox.

As previously stated, the chickenpox vaccine contains gelatin and the antibiotic neomycin. If your child is allergic to these components, she may not be eligible for the chickenpox vaccine.

Finally, there is a small but real possibility of getting shingles after receiving the chickenpox vaccine. The risk is estimated at 2 out of 100,000 doses of the chickenpox vaccine. Compared to the chance of shingles after a natural chickenpox infection, which is estimated to be 68 out of 100,000 infections, the risk of shingles after vaccination is much lower. After vaccination, shingles can appear anytime between a month and up to a few years later. Just like the "natural" shingles caused by a typical chickenpox infection, the vaccine-induced shingles is also contagious.

CHAPTER 15

The Hepatitis A Vaccine

The hepatitis A vaccine has very minimal side effects, and it has not been implicated in any controversy. However, the hepatitis A infection is also a relatively mild disease. Children rarely die from this type of hepatitis, and most children do not even need to be hospitalized. Nevertheless, hepatitis A is notorious for causing community-wide outbreaks. It can be a costly disease, and it places a tremendous financial burden on community-health resources.

Introduction

The hepatitis A vaccine is one of the newer additions to the current childhood immunization schedule. It is unique because when this vaccine first became available in 1995, it was not universally recommended for all children. Instead, it was administered in communities where hepatitis A was most common. Hepatitis A infections generally occur in outbreaks, and there are certain parts of the country that have more frequent outbreaks than others. Typically, hepatitis A is more common in states with a greater immigrant population.

When the hepatitis A vaccine was first introduced, it was recommended for children older than two years. In 2006, the age limit was lowered to twelve months so young children could be protected at an earlier age.

A combination vaccine that contains components for both the hepatitis A and hepatitis B viruses is available. This combination vaccine is administered three times—at birth, at the first month of life, and finally at six months of age.

⁉ Question

Since hepatitis A is not a life-threatening infection, how can one justify administering this vaccine to all children?
Even though hepatitis A infection is not fatal, it can still make your child very sick—sometimes requiring hospitalization for more than a week. The pain and suffering, not to mention the medical bills, are enough reason to prevent this infection.

The hepatitis A vaccine works incredibly well, but it takes approximately four weeks after the injection before the vaccine takes protective effect. Even after receiving the first dose, the vaccine protects 100 percent of the children. The second dose of the vaccine is given at least six months later to boost the immune system so the immunity can last a lifetime. If your child does not get the second dose of the hepatitis A vaccine six months after the initial dose, the second dose can be given any time after the first dose. A long interval between the two doses does not interfere with how well the vaccine works.

Hepatitis A Infection

Hepatitis A is an infection caused by a virus. This virus primarily attacks the liver, and the severity of the illness can vary quite a bit between individuals. Hepatitis A infection affects mostly children, but it can affect adults if adults travel to other parts of the world. An estimated 1.5 million people get sick from this infection each year. In many countries, close to 100 percent of the nation's population has been infected. While babies and toddlers are likely not to get sick at all when they catch this bug, older children can become so ill that they need to be hospitalized for more than a week from vomiting and dehydration.

 Fact

> Since hepatitis A infection is so common in many parts of the world, the hepatitis A vaccine is not recommended for children in developing countries. Most children in those countries are already immune to hepatitis A by the time the vaccine is scheduled to be given at age twelve months.

Ironically, outbreaks of hepatitis A only tend to happen in developed countries with good sanitation and hygiene practices. This is because almost all children from developing countries have already been exposed to hepatitis A at a very young age, so they are already immune to the infection by the time they enter school. The distribution of hepatitis A means that fecal contamination of food is very common in most parts of the world except for the United States, Canada, Japan, Western Europe, Australia, and New Zealand.

The initial illness caused by hepatitis A is indistinguishable from the illness caused by hepatitis B or hepatitis C. The only way to confirm the diagnosis is through a blood test, but the result of this test may take many days to become available. Fortunately, you can only get sick from hepatitis A once in your life. After one infection, you are immune for life.

The hepatitis A virus can survive outside of the human body for long periods of time, from weeks to months. This hardy germ can stay viable in stools that have been expelled from the body, so in places where human feces is used as natural fertilizer, contaminated vegetables and fruits can be an important source of transmission.

Hepatitis A can be challenging to diagnose. Some people who have evidence of infection from the blood test in fact do not have a current bout of hepatitis A infection. Unless you are experiencing symptoms suggestive of hepatitis, you should not get a blood test to check for hepatitis A.

Symptoms of Hepatitis A

Symptoms of a Hepatitis A inflection include:

- Fatigue
- Fever
- Sore muscles
- Headache
- Nausea
- Loss of appetite
- Pain on the right side of the body (where the liver is located)
- Yellowing of the skin and eyes (jaundice)
- Dark urine
- Diarrhea

How Does One Catch It?

Community outbreaks contribute to more than half of all hepatitis A infections. Transmission between children and then to their adult caregivers is the primary way this infection is passed within a community. An infected person sheds the virus in the stool. Even though the virus has been found in human saliva, confirmed transmission through saliva has never been proven.

Contaminated foods and direct personal contact by infected people with poor hygiene make up the majority of the means of transmission, even though it is possible to be transmitted by blood transfusion and also by sexual intercourse. Eating raw meat or undercooked meat increases the risk of catching hepatitis A. Thorough cooking in high temperature should kill any hepatitis A virus in contaminated foods.

A person infected with hepatitis A starts spreading the virus two weeks before he starts feeling sick. Even though this is the most contagious period during the infection, the person has no idea that he is shedding the virus and spreading it to others because he does not feel sick at all. In addition, anyone who gets sick from him would not feel any ill effects until a month later.

 Alert

The virus is shed in the feces of the infected person and then transmitted to another person from the contaminated hands of the sick person. If everyone, including young children, had good hygiene practices and frequent hand washing, the hepatitis A virus would never have a chance to start an outbreak in a community.

This long incubation period for the infection makes quarantine of infected individuals tremendously difficult. Children tend to stay infectious for much longer periods of time than adults. Some children continue to spread the virus more than two months after they apparently recover from an acute hepatitis A infection.

Essential

The hepatitis A virus can only make humans sick. It is impossible to get sick from your pets and vice versa. Nevertheless, thorough hand washing after touching pets is still a good idea to prevent other infectious diseases.

How Common Is the Infection?

Hepatitis A frequently causes community-wide outbreaks, but nationwide outbreaks also occur. The last outbreak that spread through the entire country took place in 1995. In the year 2000, an estimated 143,000 infections happened in the United States. The large number makes hepatitis A the most common vaccine-preventable infection in America.

🔔 Alert

Hepatitis A is a relatively common infection in most other parts of the world. If you plan to travel to anywhere outside of the United States, Western Europe, Australia, and Japan, you should get vaccinated prior to departure. The vaccine takes at least two weeks to take effect, so you should get the vaccine as soon as you confirm you travel plans.

Adults born in the United States are less likely to be infected with hepatitis A. Only about a quarter of all American adults born in the United States have been infected with hepatitis A. This is drastically lower than foreign-born residents, where up to 70 percent of them have been infected with hepatitis A in the past.

Minority groups are more likely to be affected by hepatitis A infections. In particular, Native Americans in the United States mainland and Alaska make up the highest-risk group for contracting hepatitis A in this country. When the hepatitis A vaccine became widely available in 1995, infection rates among minorities had shown the biggest reduction in any groups of people.

How Serious Is the Infection?

Hepatitis A is a viral infection that causes inflammation of the liver. Even though it is grouped together with the other viral hepatitis infections, it is quite different from hepatitis B and hepatitis C. Unlike those other types of hepatitis, hepatitis A never causes chronic hepatitis, and therefore it does not trigger liver cancer. This characteristic of hepatitis A makes it significantly less dangerous than hepatitis B or C.

Nevertheless, most people who get sick from hepatitis A still become quite ill. The sickness usually starts suddenly, with the person feeling nauseated. Abdominal pain and vomiting are common symptoms, and the person can become jaundiced quite early on in the course of the illness. The duration of the illness usually lasts a few weeks, but more than 10 percent of people may remain ill for up to six months.

 Fact

> Even though hepatitis A is usually not fatal and does not cause chronic liver infection, it costs the United States more than $200 million in medical bills and loss of work each year.

While most people stricken with hepatitis A recover completely without suffering any long-term damage to their livers, a few of them (about .5 percent) can die from hepatitis A infection. The chance of dying from hepatitis A is significantly higher for those individuals who already have chronic liver disease. People with a history of alcohol abuse tend to suffer the most serious consequences of hepatitis A infection.

Children younger than school age tend to get less sick from hepatitis A than school-age children, and adults older than fifty seldom get sick from hepatitis A. Consequently, the hepatitis A vaccine offers the most benefit for school-age children (ages five to fourteen).

Is the Infection Treatable?

There is no treatment to get rid of the hepatitis A virus once the virus enters the body. Antibiotics are useless against viruses. There is no antiviral medication against the hepatitis A virus.

Some children with hepatitis A can become dehydrated secondary to the severe vomiting that accompanies the infection. Many of these children need to stay in the hospital to get intravenous fluid to restore the watery content in their bodies. Hospitalization for more than a week is not unusual. Fortunately, almost everyone recovers completely from hepatitis A infection without any long-lasting effects.

Components of the Hepatitis A Vaccine

The hepatitis A vaccine is made from killed hepatitis A virus. The killed virus used in the vaccine is grown in human muscle cells, and they are chemically inactivated using formaldehyde. Aluminum hydroxide is then added to the vaccine to make it better stimulate the immune system. Finally, to protect the vaccine from bacterial contamination, the preservative 2-phenoxyethanol (a type of alcohol) is added to it. The hepatitis A vaccine, like all other childhood vaccines today, contains no mercury-based preservative.

🗹 Fact

If you are worried about the use of formaldehyde in many vaccines, keep in mind that whenever you consume any alcoholic beverage, some of the alcohol is temporarily converted into formaldehyde inside your body before it is excreted by the kidneys.

Side Effects of the Hepatitis A Vaccine

Only very mild reactions have been reported after the administration of the hepatitis A vaccine. The most common reaction reported both in children and in adults after receiving the hepatitis A vaccine is soreness at the site of injection. The pain usually goes away in less than two days, and it does not require any specific treatment beside over-the-counter analgesics (such as acetaminophen or ibuprofen).

Poor appetite and fatigue have also been reported three to five days after hepatitis A vaccination, but these also resolve promptly without treatment.

Fever is not a reported side effect. If your child develops a fever after the vaccination, the fever is probably caused by something else. You should call your doctor if any fever develops, because your child may have an unrelated infection.

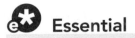 **Essential**

The hepatitis A vaccine is made from killed hepatitis A virus. Getting vaccinated for hepatitis A cannot trigger a hepatitis A infection. The dead virus is unable to cause an infection.

Finally, as with any vaccination, an allergic reaction may develop in very rare circumstances after the hepatitis A vaccination. The reaction is potentially severe, but the effect is readily reversible. If you had a serious allergic reaction to hepatitis A vaccine in the past, you should not receive the second dose of the vaccine.

CHAPTER 16

The Meningococcal Vaccine

The meningococcal vaccine can protect children from the dreaded meningitis, an infection of the brain. While there are two other types of vaccines designed to protect children from meningitis, the meningococcal vaccine is different because it prevents meningitis in adolescents as well as younger children. This vaccine is generally safe, but it has the potential for causing a rare but serious side effect. This chapter will explore all facets of the meningococcal vaccine.

Introduction

Three types of bacteria that are responsible for causing the vast majority of bacterial meningitis are *Haemophilius influenza* type b (Hib), pneumococcus, and *Neisseria meningitidis*. The Hib conjugate vaccine (discussed in Chapter 10) and the pneumococcal conjugate vaccine (discussed in Chapter 11) are designed to protect babies. The meningococcal vaccine differs from those two vaccines because it can protect children as well as adolescents.

There are two types of meningococcal vaccine. An older version of the vaccine is called the meningococcal polysaccharide vaccine. When it was first invented, it was designed to protect military personnel because meningitis outbreak is a common infectious threat to military recruits. The same vaccine first became available to the general public in 1981, and it was only recommended for children with a weakened immune system. Children without a functional spleen and children who have certain types of immune deficiencies were the main recipients of this polysaccharide vaccine.

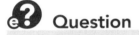 **Question**

Why are people without a functional spleen weaker at defending themselves against germs?
The spleen is a versatile organ with many functions. It is responsible for recycling worn-out blood cells from circulation, and it also screens the blood for invaders. You can think of it as a security checkpoint in the body. Without this extra layer of security, your body is vulnerable from certain bacterial invasions.

The newer meningococcal conjugate vaccine was introduced in 2005. This vaccine is primarily targeted for adolescents. Meningitis caused by meningococcus is most common in babies, but college freshmen living in dormitories make up another high-risk population who are most prone to getting the infection. When young adults from all parts of the country congregate in college dormitories in close proximity with each other, an outbreak of meningitis can spread like wildfire setting. The meningococcal conjugate vaccine was invented specifically to prevent outbreaks among college freshmen living in dorms.

Both vaccines (the older polysaccharide vaccine and the newer conjugate vaccine) can be given to children as young as two years of age, and the conjugate vaccine can be used to prevent infections for young children with weakened immune systems. However, the newer conjugate vaccine works much better than the older polysaccharide vaccine. You can think of the meningococcal conjugate vaccine as the next generation meningococcal vaccine. Over the next few years, the newer conjugate vaccine will inevitably replace its older counterpart.

The meningococcal conjugate vaccine is currently recommended for all adolescents age eleven and up. If your teen is going to college soon, this vaccine is even more important because the chance of getting meningitis is much higher for college freshmen compared to the general population. Only one dose of this vaccine is needed, and evidence shows that the vaccine retains its protective effect for more than eight years.

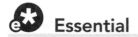 **Essential**

The effect of the older polysaccharide meningococcal vaccine does not last as long as the new conjugate vaccine. The effect wears off after a few years, especially in younger children. A booster shot was recommended every three to five years for the older vaccine. The new conjugate vaccine does not require booster doses.

Since most meningococcal infections occur in babies, the meningococcal conjugate vaccine may be recommended for babies as young as two months old in the future. In Canada, a trial of a meningococcal vaccine for babies was started in 2008.

Meningococcal Infection

You probably have heard on the news about meningitis outbreaks in college dormitories. The number of students affected is usually small in these outbreaks, but the resulting fear and panic can be widespread. In addition, for those who are directly affected, the consequences are catastrophic. Meningitis is not common among college students, but because the disease has such a high fatality rate, it is still a serious threat. The meningo-coccus bacterium causes the vast majority of meningitis among college students.

In addition to causing meningitis, the meningococcus bac-terium can also invade the bloodstream directly and cause a full-body infection. This infection can quickly lead to shock and death unless rapid treatment is instituted. There is a 40 per-cent fatality rate when meningococcal infection spreads to the whole body. Even among survivors, about 20 percent end up with permanent hearing loss, chronic seizure problems, amputa-tion of the arms or legs secondary to shock, or permanent brain damage.

There are many strains of meningococcus bacterium, but four strains are responsible for the majority of infections. The two types of meningococcal vaccines—the polysaccharide vaccine and the conjugate vaccine—both protect against only the four strains, so these vaccines do not offer complete protection from meningococ-cal infections.

Symptoms of the Meningococcal Infection

Symptoms of a meningoccal infection include:

- Irritability
- Fatigue
- Nausea and vomiting
- Head and neck pain
- Weakness
- Fever
- Chills
- Muscle pain
- Skin rash that starts as small red rash and can progress into larger red or purple lesions
- Difficulty breathing
- Coma

How Does One Catch It?

The meningococcus bacterium spreads in small droplets that are suspended in air. You can catch it by breathing the contaminated air or by touching the droplets on your hands and transferring the droplets into the nose or mouth. It can also pass from person to person through kissing or shared utensils.

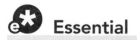 **Essential**

> Hand washing is one of the most effective ways to avoid catching germs, but many germs, including meningococcus, can be transmitted in the air as well. Even wearing a mask does not prevent transmission of meningitis effectively.

The strange thing about the meningococcus bacterium is that it can stay in some people's nose and mouth without making them sick. This is the most common way of transmission—passage of the bacteria from healthy people to others. Why this bacterium just sits in some people's mouth and causes no ill effects while causing life-threatening infection in others is unclear. Studies estimate that 10 to 25 percent of healthy people harbor this bacterium in their bodies. This is the reason why it is impossible to quarantine a meningococcal outbreak.

How Common Is the Infection?

Meningococcal infections are not common, but people die from it during most outbreaks. In 2002, a massive outbreak occurred in central Africa that sickened 13,000 people and killed 1,500. There have been sporadic outbreaks in the United States, especially in college dormitories. Over 3,000 cases of meningococcal infection were reported annually in the United States, most of which came from ten to fifteen outbreaks in various parts of the country. Ten to

15 percent of the infected people end up dying from the infection, despite prompt and appropriate treatment with antibiotics and other medications.

Meningitis caused by meningococcus used to make up only a small percentage of bacterial meningitis, but since the Hib and pneumococcal conjugate vaccines are working so well to prevent these other causes of meningitis in children, meningococcal meningitis is fast becoming the most common cause of meningitis in children.

Meningitis is most common in the winter season, and young infants are most commonly affected. The meningococcus bacterium is unique because it is the only type of bacterium that is capable of causing outbreaks of meningitis. Other bacterial meningitis usually does not involve outbreaks.

How Serious Is the Infection?

Meningococcal infection is extremely serious. Five to 10 percent of people with the infection ultimately succumb to the illness, and death usually occurs in less than two days. Since the infection spreads through the body so quickly, it is not uncommon for the infection to be overwhelming by the time the patient makes it to a hospital.

Even among the survivors, permanent brain damage, seizure problems, hearing loss, and amputation of the arms and legs are common complications after a meningococcal infection. Only a lucky few escape this dangerous infection completely unscathed.

Is the Infection Treatable?

Meningococcal infection can be treated with many different kinds of antibiotics. If treatment is instituted promptly, fatalities and long-term complications can be reduced. The tricky part is that when meningitis strikes, it resembles a bad case of the flu. By the time the diagnosis is made because of a deteriorating condition, the patient may already be very ill and treatment may not work to push back the infection.

Patients diagnosed with meningococcal infection are always hospitalized, and most, if not all, stay in the intensive care unit. In addition to antibiotics, intravenous fluid and blood pressure medications are used to treat shock when the infection becomes wide spread in the body. Surgery to remove dead limbs is sometimes necessary because the low blood pressure and clamping down of the blood vessels associated with this infection often cut off blood supply to the extremities, causing the affected limb to turn black and die. Hospitalization for more than ten days is typical for this serious infection.

Components of the Meningococcal Vaccine

The meningococcal conjugate vaccine is made from the sugar coating of the bacteria *Neisseria meningitidis*, the germ that is responsible for causing meningitis in adolescents. The chemical from the outer surface of the bacterium is extracted and purified, and it is then connected (conjugated) to the protein made by the diphtheria bacterium. The conjugation process is necessary because the protein from diphtheria alerts the immune system to the presence of the meningococcal coating much better than the sugar coating alone.

The vaccine also contains a small amount of formaldehyde (used to deactivate the protein from diphtheria bacterium). The vaccine does not contain any preservative or antibiotics. There is no trace of any animal tissue in this vaccine because both meningococcus and diphtheria are bacteria, and they do not need to be grown inside another cell to be produced in the laboratory.

Side Effects of the Meningococcal Vaccine

The meningococcal conjugate vaccine causes relatively few side effects for the vast majority of people getting this vaccine. Pain at the injection site is a common reaction after vaccination, as well as mild irritability and headache (as reported by older children). Injection-site pain and swelling occurred in 45 percent and 17 percent of people, respectively. Fever occurred in about 5 percent of individuals after receiving the meningococcal vaccine.

 Alert

If you experienced Guillain Barré Syndrome in the past, you should not receive the meningococcal vaccine as it may trigger the same reaction again. Definitely tell your doctor about this reaction if you have a history of Guillain Barré Syndrome.

Even though the meningococcal vaccine is very safe most of the time, a few people have come down with a rare but serious condition called Guillain Barré Syndrome after getting the meningococcal vaccine. While Guillain Barré Syndrome is rare and other illnesses can trigger this reaction, people who receive the meningococcal vaccine seem to have a slightly greater chance of getting this reaction after the shot. About one in a million people may experience this reaction after receiving this vaccine. For additional discussion on Guillain Barré Syndrome, please refer to Chapter 3 regarding vaccine reactions.

Guillain Barré Syndrome is when one's own immune system attacks the nerves in the spinal cord. It can cause loss of sensation and paralysis of the arms, legs, and face. The paralysis is usually temporary, but it can last many weeks to months. More than 85 percent of the people with Guillain Barré Syndrome recover completely, but some have residual weakness in their extremities. Very few people with Guillain Barré Syndrome die from the reaction because supportive treatments are available to assist breathing during the worst phase of the reaction.

Understandably, knowing the possibility of paralysis that could be caused by this vaccine could make you think twice about vaccinating your child with it. On the other hand, the threat of meningitis is also very real in adolescents. As mentioned before, 10 to 25 percent of healthy people harbor this bacterium and can pass it to others. It is impossible to predict who might fall ill next. Keep in mind that more than 2,500 people are infected by meningococcus annually in the United States, while the chance of getting Guillain Barré Syndrome from the vaccine is one in a million. Deciding whether to get the vaccine is a matter of comparing the odds.

CHAPTER 17

The HPV Vaccine

The HPV vaccine is one of the newest additions to the immunization schedule. It has stirred some controversy because many parents feel uneasy about vaccinating their children against a sexually transmitted disease at a young age. Urban legend also claims that the HPV vaccine can actually cause cancer instead of preventing it. This chapter will clarify the indication for the vaccine, explain how this vaccine works, and bust any myths that are circulating about this vaccine.

Introduction

In October 2008, Dr. Harald zur Hausen won the Nobel Prize in Medicine for discovering the human papilloma virus (HPV) and ascertaining the role of this virus in causing cervical cancer. Cervical cancer is the second most common cancer in women. Dr. zur Hausen's discovery paved the way for development of the first vaccine that can prevent cervical cancer. This vaccine has the potential for saving millions of lives around the world.

The HPV vaccine became available to the general public in 2006, after undergoing extensive test to ensure its safety. More than 10,000 people received the HPV vaccine during its testing phase and experienced no side effects other than soreness of the arm at the injection site. Millions of doses of this vaccine have been administered since, and no serious side effects have been seen.

The HPV vaccine is recommended for all women age nine to twenty-six. The reason why the vaccine is recommended to young girls is because the vaccine doesn't work well after the first sexual encounter. Even though your daughter is not going to have sex until much later, it is important to protect her early. Just like the rubella vaccine is designed to prevent congenital rubella syndrome, which does not occur until the girl becomes pregnant, the HPV vaccine is given at an early age to prevent catastrophe later in life.

Question

Since girls can get the HPV infection from infected boys, why aren't boys immunized against the infection as well?
The HPV vaccine had only been tested in girls, so it is not known whether the vaccine is safe for boys. There is plan to eventually vaccinate boys with the HPV vaccine in the future, once it has been tested in boys.

To fully benefit from the HPV vaccine, it is necessary to get three doses. The vaccine is injected into the muscle, like most vaccines. The first two doses of the vaccine must be separated by at least two months, and the third dose must be given at least six months after the initial dose. The minimum interval between the second and the third dose is three months, assuming the third dose is given at least six months after the initial dose. An earlier dose of the vaccine never expires, which means as long as you get a total of three doses, the vaccines do not need to be given at exactly two- and four-month intervals.

Even though this vaccine was primarily invented to prevent cancer, the HPV vaccine also prevents genital warts. In fact, the vaccine is even more effective at preventing genital warts than preventing cervical cancer. While genital warts are not life threatening, they are painful, embarrassing, and could be debilitating.

It is important to understand that while this vaccine works very well, it does not prevent all the strains of the HPV that can cause cancer and warts. Therefore, it is still important to practice safe sex. It is possible to get both cervical cancer and genital warts even after completing the vaccine series, and it remains important to get an annual Pap smear to screen for cervical cancer.

Many parents think this vaccine is not necessary because their daughter is only going to have one sexual partner. Premarital sex is not condoned in many households. However, it is possible to become infected with HPV even if a woman only has one sexual partner in her entire lifetime. Many men who are infected with HPV do not show any symptoms or signs of genital warts, yet they can still pass the infection to their sexual partner.

Human Papilloma Virus

In addition to causing cervical cancer, HPV is also the most common cause of warts on the skin in children. The infection is extremely common and was estimated to cause more than 6 million infections in Americans in the year 2000.

 Fact

HPV is not unique in the respect that an infection can lead to cancer. Other viruses can also cause cancer in humans. The hepatitis B virus can cause liver cancer, HIV can cause a rare type of skin cancer, and the Epstein-Barr virus can cause throat cancer and a certain type of lymphoma.

There are more than 100 strains of human papilloma virus. The strains are quite distinct, and each specializes in a particular type of infection. Some types are responsible for causing common warts on the hands and feet of children, while other strains cause genital warts and cervical cancer. Even though common warts are contagious, they tend to be a lot less contagious than genital warts.

While most HPV infection does not lead to cancer, the most serious complication from the infection is, of course, cervical cancer. Almost all cervical cancers are triggered by HPV infection. Cervical cancer can usually be detected early if women have routine annual Pap smear screening, and this is the reason why most cervical cancers are not fatal. However, in the absence of regular screening, cervical cancer can spread undetected to other parts of the body and become life threatening.

Question

Can the HPV vaccine help prevent cervical cancer for women who have already had sexual intercourse?
Even though the HPV vaccine works best for girls who have never had sexual intercourse, it can still benefit those who are already sexually active. The later this vaccine is given after the first sexual encounter, the less helpful it is.

Symptoms of HPV

Most people that contract HPV don't know that they have it because there are often few visible symptoms. Often in females HPV is not discovered until the patient gets an abnormal result on a routine pap smear. A further test is then needed to diagnose if the HPV virus is present.

An individual who has contracted HPV may feel and appear perfectly healthy. The symptoms of the HPV virus include:

- Genital warts in, around, and on the vagina, penis, scrotum, and anus (Often the warts are cauliflower shaped)

- Cervical cancer
- Some strains of HPV can also cause common warts on other areas of the body such as the hands and feet

The genital warts associated with HPV can show up weeks or even months after sexual contact with a person infected with the HPV virus. The person may not even know he or she is infected and is responsible for the transmission.

How Does One Catch It?

HPV is transmitted by direct skin-to-skin contact. A regular wart on the skin may result from casual contact, but genital warts are generally acquired during sexual activities.

 Alert

It is crucial to understand that protected sexual intercourse (that is, using condoms or other barrier methods) does not prevent the HPV infection. Direct skin-to-skin contact anywhere on the body allows transmission of this virus.

An infected person may have no visible wart on the skin or the genital area to remain contagious. Just because your sexual partner does not have any warts does not mean that he cannot transmit genital warts to you.

A mother infected with genital warts can pass the infection to her newly born baby during labor and delivery. This condition can result in one of the most devastating conditions in children. Babies who catch the virus at birth develop warts in their throats, which require surgical removal every few weeks for more than a decade. Some children end up having more than fifty operations for this condition before the age of ten. If you have a history of genital warts and become pregnant, your baby may end up paying the price for the infection.

How Common Is the Infection?

HPV is the most common sexually transmitted disease in the United States. An estimated 20 million Americans are infected with the virus, and the infection is particularly common among young adults.

 Fact

More than 40 percent of women between the ages of twenty to twenty-four are infected with HPV. They can pass on the infection to their sexual partners unknowingly, because many of them would not have any visible lesions in the genital area.

Four thousand women die from cervical cancer each year in the United States, and this trend is increasing due to the widespread HPV infection in this country.

How Serious Is the Infection?

HPV infection is responsible for causing cervical cancer, but what is cervical cancer? Cervical cancer occurs when cells in the cervix (the "mouth" of the uterus, found at the end of the vagina) become infected with HPV and start multiplying unregulated. The tumor from cervical cancer grows very slowly, and the person with this type of cancer experiences no symptoms until the tumor has extensively invaded the surrounding tissue. Vaginal bleeding may occur late in the course of the disease.

If cervical cancer is detected early, it can be readily treated with surgery, but chemotherapy and radiation treatment are necessary if the cancer is already wide spread by the time it is diagnosed.

The mortality rate is not high, but close to 4,000 people still died from cervical cancer in 2008 because this cancer is so common.

Is the Infection Treatable?

The HPV infection itself is not treatable with any antibiotics or antiviral medications. The best way to avoid the infection is through prevention. Complete lifelong abstinence is a sure way to avoid genital warts and cervical cancer. Studies have shown that cervical cancer is extremely rare among nuns.

While genital warts are not fatal, they can still be debilitating. Genital warts can be painful, and the growth can become quite large without treatment. The warts look like cauliflower in the genital area in both men and women. No effective treatment is currently available to prevent the recurrence of the warts, and the treatment itself is painful. Most commonly, an acid is used to cause a chemical burn to destroy the wart. Alternatively, a freezing agent (most commonly liquid nitrogen) can be used to cause localized frostbite to the wart to get rid of the lesion.

Cervical cancer, on the other hand, is treatable with surgery, chemotherapy, and radiation. While these treatment options may not be pleasant, they often offer good results with the possibility of a cure. The earlier cervical cancer is detected, the better the prognosis. It is extremely important for all women to get an annual Pap smear screening. The only group of people who don't require screening are those who never had any sexual contact and never plan to do so. Monogamy, contrary to common belief, does not protect you from HPV infection.

Components of the HPV Vaccine

The HPV vaccine is different from most other vaccines because the viral components in the vaccine are not derived from the actual virus itself. The ingredients are made in the laboratory by bioengineering, so the vaccine is completely devoid of whole viral particles. Since the vaccine does not contain any viral parts, it is impossible for the vaccine to cause HPV infection.

The HPV vaccine does not contain thimerosal, and this mercury-based preservative is never used during the vaccine manufacturing process.

Side Effects of the HPV Vaccine

More than 16 million doses of the HPV vaccine have been given, and the number of side effects reported is small compared to most other vaccines. The HPV vaccine is one of the few vaccines that does not cause any fever, but it can cause significant soreness at the site of injection for most people. Since this is a temporary side effect that is more of a nuisance than a threat, most people accept the discomfort without worrying about it too much.

 Alert

The HPV vaccine has not been tested in pregnant women, so you should not get this vaccine if you are pregnant. However, this vaccine has not been reported to be responsible for any birth defects if given to pregnant women.

A year after the HPV vaccine became widely available, reports started surfacing that several people died after the vaccine. So far, ten confirmed deaths, which occurred soon after the HPV vaccination, have been investigated by the CDC. The investigation revealed that the deaths were results of motor vehicle accidents or other unrelated reasons, and the vaccine was not responsible for the deaths. However, the damage to the reputation of the vaccine was done. Many parents heard about this report of deaths following vaccination on the evening news, but there was no clarification of the circumstances of deaths at the time. Now many parents hesitate to vaccinate their children.

You may also hesitate to vaccinate your daughter at such a young age against a sexually transmitted disease. While it is perfectly fine to wait, just don't wait too long. It takes at least six months to complete this vaccine series, and most adolescent girls do not get all three doses for more than two years due to missed appointments. It is all too easy to forget about an appointment scheduled six months in advance with a busy schedule.

CHAPTER 18

The Flu Vaccine

The flu vaccine is unusual because it is recommended for children and adults alike. It also differs from other vaccines in that a different flu vaccine is made each year, and getting the flu shot last year doesn't mean you will be protected this year. Many people are worried about getting the flu vaccine because they think the vaccine will make them come down with the flu. This chapter will clarify all of your questions and allow you to make the best decision for you and your family.

Introduction

In some ways, the flu vaccine is an optional vaccine because it is not required for any school admission or work attendance. Consequently, only a small percentage of the population typically gets vaccinated each year. Due to the low vaccination rate, the vaccine manufacturers do not even make enough vaccine each year for every vaccine-eligible person. During the year when vaccine shortage is not an issue, millions of doses of the flu vaccine are routinely destroyed because they are unused by the end of the flu season.

The reason why last year's flu vaccine is no good for the current year is that each year the types of flu virus that circulate are different from the year before. This is the reason why people may catch the flu year after year if they are not vaccinated. The flu virus is very tricky. Different strains of the virus take turns in causing outbreaks each winter, so even if everyone's immune system remembers the virus that caused the flu from years ago, a different strain can still sneak past your immune defenses and wreak havoc on your body.

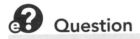

Question

Since the flu vaccine cannot be given to everyone, how do you know whether you or your child needs the flu vaccine?
The flu vaccine is especially recommended for children less than eighteen years old (but older than six months) and for adults older than fifty. In addition, people with asthma, heart problems, or weakened immune systems should get vaccinated. Household members of those who are at risk should be immunized as well.

The constantly changing nature of the flu virus is also the reason why a new flu vaccine must be made each year. Last year's flu vaccine would not work very well for the current flu season. On June 30 of each year, the leftover flu vaccines from the year before are all destroyed so a new batch can be made for the following flu season. This also means that if you got the flu shot last year, you'll have to get it again this year to stay protected.

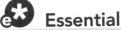

Essential

It takes the flu vaccine two weeks to get your immune system ready to fight off the flu virus. This means that if you received the flu vaccine two weeks ago, you can still catch the flu until two weeks after the shot. This is why you need to get vaccinated as early as possible in the flu season.

The changing flu virus also makes the production of the flu vaccine very challenging. In order to make the vaccine that works for each particular flu season, scientists must predict before the flu season starts which strains of the flu virus will cause outbreaks. Scientists and doctors can make educated guesses from patterns of previous flu outbreaks and trends of infection from years before. Nevertheless, the prediction is not always perfect. If the scientists guess incorrectly, the flu vaccine will not work as well.

 Fact

In 2003, the flu vaccine manufacturer Wyeth had to destroy more than 6 million doses of the flu vaccine because of weak demand. The company lost more than $30 million that year and was forced out of the flu vaccine business for the following year. A massive vaccine shortage ensued in 2004.

You may wonder why scientists cannot wait until the beginning of the flu season to see which flu strains are circulating before making the flu vaccine. The problem is that it takes six months to produce the flu vaccine. If scientists wait until the beginning of the flu season to make the vaccines, by the time the vaccines are made available, the flu season would be over. The vaccine would be quite useless by then.

Fortunately, each flu vaccine is able to protect against three flu strains. So even if scientists guess wrong on two out of three strains, the vaccine would still protect some individuals from getting sick. In a good year, the flu vaccine works perfectly because the scientists predict all three of the flu strains that are responsible for the flu season.

The difficult process of making the flu vaccine is also the reason why there were massive vaccine shortages in the past. Vaccine-making companies usually have to write off huge financial losses each year because of weak demand for the vaccine and the mandatory destruction of a large number of the vaccines at the end of the flu season. Consequently, many companies simply stopped making the flu vaccine.

Due to these various limitations of the flu vaccine, scientists are working hard at inventing a flu vaccine that works for all strains of the flu virus. Once this all-purpose flu vaccine becomes available in the future, throwing away unused vaccines will not be necessary anymore.

There are two types of the flu vaccine. The injectable form of the vaccine is approved for children older than six months, and the nasal spray flu vaccine (trade name FluMist) is approved for children older than two years of age. Children less than nine years old getting the flu vaccine for the first time in their lives need to receive two doses of the vaccine to be fully protected. The two doses of the flu vaccine need to be separated by least four weeks.

Question

Can pregnant women get the flu shot during the first trimester of pregnancy?
The injectable form of the flu vaccine (the vaccine that contains killed flu virus) is safe for pregnant women. In fact, a 2008 study published in the *New England Journal of Medicine* demonstrated that babies born to mothers who had the flu shot during pregnancy get sick less often.

Influenza Infection

The flu, like many other infections, tends to make some people sicker than others. Those who are most vulnerable include the very young, the very old, people with heart and lung problems, and those with impaired immune systems. For most healthy people, having the flu is still a miserable experience, but at least it is not life threatening.

Symptoms of the flu usually start suddenly, with characteristic high fever, aches and pains, sore throat, red eyes, and general fatigue. It simply sucks the energy out of your body. These symptoms usually improve after three to four days, and a nasty cough starts later in the course. The cough can last for more than two weeks.

For those less fortunate, complications from the flu infection can result in pneumonia, sinus infection, infection of the brain, and even death. These serious problems are not common in young adults, but even healthy individuals are not entirely immune to these complications. During the flu pandemic of 1918, 40 million people died, including many healthy adults.

📢 Alert

In the flu season that ended in 2008, seventy-two children died from the flu. The season ended in May 2008. Information for the 2008–2009 flu season was not available at the time this book was written.

You may have heard about the flu pandemic in the news, especially the swine flu pandemic in early 2009. A global pandemic occurs when the flu virus changes itself so much that it is almost transformed to an entirely new virus. The danger of this transformation is twofold. For one, the new flu virus becomes so different that very few people's immune systems are prepared to fight off such an infection. Typically, if you got sick from the flu in past years, your body is going to be somewhat immune to the flu in the future. That's because the different strains of flu virus still share some similarities, so a small degree of immunity persists after each infection.

However, when the flu virus mutates drastically, it becomes an entirely new beast. Your immune system cannot recognize the mutant virus at all, so you are completely vulnerable to the infection.

This is also true for everyone else in the world. This is only one of the reasons why a flu pandemic is so deadly. The virus is a new evil that no one has ever seen before. By the time the human immune system detects the new virus, it is often too late.

Another reason why a mutated virus is dangerous is that the new flu may be more aggressive and cause more life-threatening problems than the typical flu virus. The 1918 flu was characterized by massive bleeding from internal organs and a high rate of complication due to bacterial pneumonia. The virus was so virulent that even healthy adults perished from the flu.

It is impossible to predict when the next global flu pandemic may occur. The mutant flu virus frequently originates from an existing flu virus that affects primarily animals. You probably heard of the bird flu and more recently the swine flu. Bird flu hasn't reached pandemic status, but swine flu was declared a pandemic by the World Health Organization in June 2009.

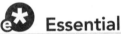 **Essential**

Other types of the flu virus that affect animals can occasionally make humans sick. You may have heard of the bird flu (or avian flu), the swine flu, and the canine flu virus. These viruses usually do not infect humans, but when they do, they are capable of causing a massive worldwide outbreak that can kill millions of people.

Symptoms of the Flu

Symptoms of the flu include:

- Fever (usually high)
- Muscle and joint aches
- Weakness and extreme tiredness
- Flushed skin
- Watery eyes

- Headache
- Cough
- Sore throat
- Runny nose
- Nasal congestion
- Loss of appetite
- Chills

The following is the story of a real family during the 1918 flu pandemic. It is reproduced with permission from the CDC's *Pandemic Flu Storybook* (2008, from *www.pandemicflu.gov/storybook*).

Storyteller: Debbie Crane

Location: North Carolina

When I was just learning to read, I prided myself on reading anything that presented itself. It was on a late spring day in 1966 when I found myself reading the tombstones in a small mountainside cemetery in western North Carolina. I had gone to the cemetery with my mother, Jessie Crane, and my grandmother, Edna Breedlove Clampitt. I remember scampering up to my mother and asking her why several of the tombstones seemed to have the same date of death. She told me to ask my grandmother that question. I did, and my grandmother told me the story of her family and the flu that swept across the country almost a half century before our journey to the cemetery.

In the late fall of 1918, Edna and her family (her pregnant mother, dad, and five siblings) were living in a cabin in Swain County, North Carolina. Even today, Swain County is pretty much disconnected from the rest of the world. It is a long two-hour drive from Asheville, North Carolina. In 1918, it was even more disconnected. No one there had heard about the flu. They pretty much lived their own lives farming, raising families, and "praising the Lord."

One of my grandmother's brothers, Wade Breedlove, had joined the army. The family was thrilled when he came home for a visit in November. They "put the big pot in the little pot" for his visit, which means that they cooked special meals and everyone came to visit. No one knew that their brother had brought an untimely death to visit. He became ill shortly after he returned to base, but he survived.

The rest of the family wasn't so lucky. By mid-December, the whole family was terribly ill. They ached. Their throats hurt. They coughed and coughed. My great-grandmother, Ida Mae Breedlove, gave birth even as she lay sick. My grandmother described one terrible night when the whole family sounded as if they were all drowning. In the morning, Ida and two-year old Woodrow were dead. The newborn, named Paul, died days later. My grandmother was never sure if it was the flu that killed him, or if he simply starved to death in a household where everyone was just too weak to take care of him.

Eventually, the rest of the family got better and moved on as best as they could without the strong mountain woman who had been their center. Until the day she died, at age ninety-three, my Grandma Clampitt never remembered being this ill again. She was a woman of deep personal faith who recalled a moment near Christmas that year when she thought she saw an angel. That moment gave her the will to go on.

How Does One Catch It?

There are three ways you can catch the flu virus. If a sick person sneezes or coughs, the virus becomes suspended in the air, and you can breathe it in. You can also contract it by touching a contaminated object. If an object is contaminated by the secretion of a sick person (such as nasal discharge or saliva), it becomes a source of infection. Finally, direct contact of the secretion from a sick person will get you sick as well.

🔔 Alert

School-age children are the main vectors for the flu during an outbreak. Their immune system is weaker than that of an adult, and their poor hygiene practice makes transmission easy. Children get sick from their peers at school and bring the infection home to everyone else.

The flu is one of the most contagious infections. It spreads extremely rapidly within a household, but an outbreak also travels swiftly through any community. Even with a complete shutdown of air travel, a flu pandemic can still race through the globe in a matter of months. It is impossible to quarantine the infection because affected individuals become contagious a day before the onset of any symptoms.

How Common Is the Infection?

The flu is extremely common for children. An estimated 10 to 40 percent of healthy children catch the flu each year, and about 1 percent of them need to stay in the hospital due to the gravity of the illness.

Pandemic flu tends to occur in ten-year cycles. During the twentieth century, three flu pandemics swept around the globe, occurring in 1918, 1957, and again in 1968.

How Serious Is the Infection?

While most children and healthy adults recover from the flu without suffering any long-term effects, children less than five years and people older than sixty-five are much more likely to experience serious illness and deaths. Common complications from the flu include pneumonia, ear infection, muscle breakdown, and dehydration. Life-threatening problems, including swelling of the brain and coma, can occur, but they are less common.

During a flu pandemic, the circulating flu virus is typically much more aggressive. In some situations, more than half will die from the infection.

Is the Infection Treatable?

There are medications to fight the flu virus, but they are not very effective. At most, the medication can reduce the duration of the illness by one day. In addition, the medication must be given within the first forty-eight hours of the illness, otherwise it is completely useless. Currently these medications are only recommended for people with weakened immune systems.

Even though antibiotics are not useful for treating the flu directly, they are often used to treat bacterial complication from the flu infection. Pneumonia, sinus infection, and ear infection can be managed with antibiotics.

Types of Flu Vaccine

The flu vaccine, like the polio vaccine in the past, is available in two main varieties. A vaccine that is made from killed virus is available in an injectable form, and a vaccine that is made from weakened live virus is available in the form of a nasal spray. These two types of vaccine work equally well.

The Flu Shot

The injectable form of the flu vaccine is made from killed flu virus. It is recommended for children down to age six months. Anyone who is eligible for the flu vaccine can request it from his or her doctor once the flu vaccine becomes available each winter season (usually in September or October).

You can safely receive the injectable form of the flu vaccine even if you are pregnant. You should not get the live flu vaccine (the nasal vaccine) during pregnancy.

The Nasal Spray Flu Vaccine

A live flu vaccine is available in the form of a nasal spray. This virus contains weakened but living flu virus, so the virus from the vaccine can actually multiply in the body after the vaccine is administered. However, the weakened virus in the vaccine cannot cause a full-blown flu infection.

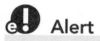 **Alert**

The nasal flu vaccine that contains live virus (FluMist) can trigger an asthma attack for people with asthma. If you or your child has asthma, the injectable killed flu vaccine should be used.

The live flu vaccine cannot be given to children younger than two years or pregnant women. This live vaccine is not as widely available as the injectable form of the killed flu vaccine.

How Well Do Flu Vaccines Work?

The effectiveness of the flu vaccine depends on a lot of factors. As was mentioned previously, scientists have to predict the strains of the flu virus each year to tailor the annual vaccine. If the prediction is accurate, the flu vaccine for that year works exceptionally well. However, if the prediction is wrong, the usefulness of the flu vaccine is more limited.

 Alert

Keep in mind that the flu vaccine can only protect you from the flu, not the common cold. There is no vaccine available for the common cold, and it is entirely possible to get sick from a cold even if you have gotten the flu vaccine.

In addition, the age of the person receiving the flu vaccine also influences how well the vaccine works. Older individuals generally respond more weakly to the vaccine than younger, healthy people. At the same time, older people are more vulnerable to having serious complications from the flu virus. Even though the flu vaccine tends to work less well in older people, they still should get vaccinated because there is no better alternative in preventing the flu.

Components of the Flu Vaccine

The virus grown in the chicken egg is purified and killed before it is made into a vaccine, but the purification process isn't perfect. A very small amount of chicken egg tissue is still present in the flu vaccine. This is the reason why you should not get the flu vaccine if you know you have severe allergy to eggs.

 Fact

Viruses, unlike bacteria, cannot live and reproduce outside of another animal's cell. To grow them during the vaccine manufacturing process, the tissue from some animal must be used. For the flu vaccine, the virus is grown in a chicken egg.

Flu vaccines designed for children do not contain the mercury preservative thimerosal, but some flu vaccines for adults and older children may contain thimerosal. Ask your doctor specifically whether the vaccine you are getting contains this preservative if you are concerned about thimerosal safety.

Side Effects of the Flu Vaccine

Common side effects of the flu vaccine include fever, mild muscle aches, and headache. These side effects are more common if you have never had the flu before or if you are getting the flu vaccine for the first time.

Essential

Many people believe that getting the flu shot actually makes you get the flu, but this is impossible. The flu shot (the injectable form of the flu vaccine) is made from dead flu virus. Killed flu virus cannot cause an infection because the virus is already dead.

Some people experience a full-blown case of the flu right after they receive their flu shot, which often makes them hesitate to get the flu shot in the future. This happens to a lot of people. Most people do not get the flu vaccine before the flu season starts. They are motivated only after people all around them are coming down with the flu, then they hurry to the doctor's office to get their flu shot. Since it takes at least two weeks for the flu vaccine to bolster your immune system, you are completely vulnerable in the interim.

What happens to these people is that they were already exposed to the flu a day or two before they got the flu shot, and the incubation period for the flu is one to three days. So it makes sense that they soon become symptomatic after the vaccination. Naturally, it would appear that the flu vaccine made them sick, but in reality they are coming down with the flu before the flu vaccine had a chance to protect them. This is the reason why you should get vaccinated before the flu season starts.

 Alert

The safety profile and side effects of the new H1N1 flu (swine flu) vaccine is unknown at the time the manuscript of this book was prepared. Please consult your doctor for the most current information and recommendation about this vaccine.

Even though most people only experience mild reactions after the flu vaccine, two serious complications may occur after the flu vaccine. Fortunately, they are extremely rare (about a one in a million chance), but these reactions could be life threatening.

The first one is a whole-body allergic reaction to the egg component in the vaccine. This reaction is called anaphylaxis, and it causes your entire body to swell up. If the swelling is not immediately stopped with medication, it could cause your throat to collapse and you may die from asphyxiation.

The other serious problem that has been caused by the flu vaccine is Guillain Barré Syndrome. This is a condition where your own immune system goes haywire and attacks the nerves inside your spinal cord. You may lose sensation of your arms and legs and become temporarily paralyzed if you develop this problem. People rarely die from Guillain Barré Syndrome, but a few people may never regain the full use of their arms and legs. Please refer to Chapter 3 for a more in-depth discussion on these serious side effects of the flu vaccine.

Finally, certain people are at higher risk for developing serious problems after getting the flu vaccine. If you belong to the groups of people described in the following list, you should not get the flu vaccine.

- Children less than six months of age (the flu vaccine is not approved for this age group because it has never been tested for children younger than six months).
- People who have a severe allergy to chicken eggs.
- People who have had a severe reaction to a flu vaccination.
- People who developed Guillain Barré Syndrome within six weeks of getting a flu vaccine.
- People who have a moderate to severe illness with a fever (they should wait until they recover to get vaccinated).

Of course, if you still have questions about whether you are eligible for getting the flu vaccine, the best source of information is your doctor. Give her a call and make sure you have all of your questions answered satisfactorily.

CHAPTER 19

Vaccines for Specific Conditions

N ot all children are created the same, and many children with certain medical conditions require a specialized vaccination schedule or additional vaccines to protect them from illnesses. Many medical conditions, such as asthma, are quite common in children, and having asthma makes children more likely to become hospitalized from infections. This section of the book is devoted to children with special circumstances that may predispose them to certain types of infections. The modification of the standard immunization schedule for these children will be discussed in detail.

Prematurity

Due to advancements in medical technology, premature babies today usually survive to adulthood and lead healthy and productive lives. Just a few decades ago, most babies born too early died because their lungs were not ready to breathe on their own. Now there are more children who were born prematurely than ever before. While the vast majority of them do very well, some of them have problems that can persist into late childhood.

Even though premature babies are born early, it is not necessary to postpone routine childhood immunization. In fact, these babies typically have weakened immune systems and need the routine immunization even more than other babies.

The only exception to the immunization schedule for extremely premature babies (babies who are less than four pounds at birth) is that these very tiny babies should not get the hepatitis B vaccine right at birth. The hepatitis B vaccine for these very small babies should be postponed for at least a week. Studies have shown that if the hepatitis B vaccine is given too soon it does not work very well.

Premature Lungs

Babies born more than a month before their due date almost invariably have lungs that are not completely ready to breathe air immediately after birth. Of all the internal organs of a fetus, the lungs are the last to reach maturity. Normally, during the last month of gestation, the fetal lungs produce a substance that allows the lungs to fully expand almost instantly after birth, allowing the newborn baby to start breathing in oxygen right away after birth. Babies who are born early never have the chance to make this substance, so when they are born, doctors must manually pump air and oxygen into their lungs.

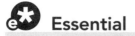 **Essential**

The substance that allows the newborn's lungs to expand right at birth is called surfactant. Surfactant is a chemical that works like soap. It reduces the surface tension of the fluid in the lungs so it does not take a lot of effort to expand the lungs and fill them with air.

Unfortunately, the lungs are not designed to have air actively pumped into them. In the process of keeping these premature babies alive, the active pumping of air into the lungs can sometimes damage the lungs. The longer these babies need aggressive help with their breathing, the more likely their lungs will be damaged.

Consequently, many premature babies, especially the ones who were born extremely early (earlier than twenty-eight weeks gestation), end up with lung damage. These babies with damaged lungs often grow up with weakened lungs, and they tend to develop wheezing later on in life. If these babies catch a cold or flu, they are likely to become extremely ill and often require many days of hospitalization.

RSV

RSV stands for "respiratory syncytial virus." The word "syncy-tial" is used to describe this virus because the virus has a tendency to make infected cells stick to each other, as if the cells are having a meeting, or syncytium.

RSV is an extremely common infection among infants. Virtu-ally every child has had this infection by the time she is three years old. Similar to the flu, most RSV infections occur during the winter months. In older children or full-term babies, RSV can cause a bad cold, but it is almost never life threatening. However, in premature babies with damaged lungs, RSV infection could be fatal.

❗ Alert

If your baby was born more than two months before the due date, ask your doctor whether he needs to get the RSV injections. The RSV injections are extremely expensive and not all hospitals or doctor's offices offer them.

RSV is passed from one person to another by contact of secre-tion. Most commonly, a tiny amount of secretion from a sick baby containing the virus is touched by a care provider, and the secre-tion is transferred to other places on the hands. The virus can stay alive on a contaminated surface for many hours. If another person (often other children or babies) touches the contaminated object, the virus is transferred to the next victim.

Since premature babies are more vulnerable to serious RSV infections, doctors routinely recommend very premature babies (usually babies born before thirty-two weeks gestation or more than two months prior to the due date) receive antibody against RSV during each winter season.

The RSV antibody is administered once a month during the entire winter season, when RSV infections are wide spread. Since the RSV antibody injection is very expensive, it is reserved for only extremely premature babies and babies with heart problems. Healthy or full-term babies are not eligible to get the RSV antibody injections.

The Flu Shot

In addition to RSV infections, the flu also poses a big threat to premature babies. For the same reasons that premature babies are more prone to getting serious problems from RSV infections, the flu can make these babies extremely ill. Premature babies with lung damage are significantly more likely to become hospitalized with the flu than healthy babies. For more information on the flu vaccine, please refer to Chapter 18.

It is recommended that premature babies receive flu shots annually, starting at six months of age. During the first flu season, these babies should get a booster flu vaccine to maximize the benefit from the flu vaccine.

Pregnancy

Vaccination during pregnancy is tricky, because the effect of the vaccine on the unborn fetus is difficult to determine. Therefore, immunization is typically postponed until the babies have been delivered or only if an infection during pregnancy poses clear harm to the mother or the fetus.

On the other hand, the immune system of a pregnant woman is significantly reduced. Being pregnant suppresses the immune system; otherwise the mother's immune system would attack and destroy the fetus because it would recognize the fetus as foreign material inside the body. Consequently, pregnant women are more prone to getting sick than before they were pregnant.

Only three vaccines are routinely recommended to women during pregnancy. They are the flu vaccine, the tetanus vaccine, and the hepatitis B vaccine. All three vaccines have been given to pregnant women for many decades, and no adverse effect on the fetus has ever been reported.

The Flu Vaccine

The flu vaccine that contains killed flu virus can be safely given to pregnant women. On the other hand, the flu vaccine that contains live but weakened flu virus should be avoided during pregnancy.

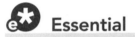 **Essential**

While mercury-based thimerosal has not been shown to cause birth defects, doctors still recommend pregnant women to get flu vaccines that do not contain this preservative. If you are pregnant, ask your doctor to make sure that a mercury-free version of the flu vaccine is ordered for you.

The rationale for giving the flu vaccine during pregnancy is that a serious case of the flu could put the lives of both the mother and the unborn child in danger. The potential risk posed by the vaccine is much smaller. Given the fact that the immune system is already weakened during pregnancy, it is prudent to bolster the immune system with the flu vaccine.

The new vaccine to protect against the novel H1N1 flu virus (the swine flu) is especially important for pregnant women, because pregnant women are a lot more likely to die from the swine flu than the general population. Many pregnant women have already perished from the swine flu, and most of them were previously healthy women.

The Tetanus Vaccine

Since tetanus is such a deadly infection, the tetanus vaccine is recommended for pregnant women. If a mother gets tetanus during pregnancy, the poison released from the tetanus bacteria could spread throughout the body and to the fetus. Both the mother and the baby are probably going to die from tetanus unless the mother is protected. It is still a better idea to get completely updated on immunization prior to getting pregnant, but as you are well aware, not all pregnancies are planned.

The Hepatitis B Vaccine

The hepatitis B vaccine is recommended even during pregnancy because hepatitis B infection in the mother could be devastating for the baby. Babies who are born to mothers with hepatitis B infection are very likely to become infected with the virus. If these babies get hepatitis from their mothers, almost all of them are going to suffer serious and chronic problem with their livers. Many of these babies who are infected ended up dying from liver failure years down the road.

Other Vaccines During Pregnancy

There are additional vaccines that have been proven to be relatively safe during pregnancy, but they are usually avoided unless the threat of an infection is imminent and the risk from complication of the infection outweighs the potential risk from vaccination. These include the pneumococcal conjugate vaccine (Chapter 11) and the hepatitis A vaccine (Chapter 15).

Certain vaccines should almost always be avoided during pregnancy, especially any vaccines that contain live virus. The MMR (measles, mumps, rubella) vaccine (Chapter 13) and the chickenpox vaccine (Chapter 14) are among the common vaccines that contain live viruses. If you are not up-to-date on these vaccines during pregnancy, you should consider getting these vaccines after you deliver your baby.

Asthma

Asthma is the most common chronic medical condition affecting children today. Nearly 5 million children have asthma in the United States, and it is a constant threat to their well-being.

Asthma is a type of allergic condition in which the lungs are hypersensitive to irritants. Children with asthma are especially susceptible to infections involving the nose, mouth, and the rest of the lungs. A child without asthma may catch a cold and recover without suffering any significant problems, but children with asthma can get extremely ill and even die if they become infected by the same virus.

 Alert

> There are two forms of the flu vaccine. The most common form comes in an injectable vaccine, and it contains killed flu virus. This is the vaccine recommended for children with asthma. Children with wheezing should not get the nasal spray form of the flu vaccine, which contains live flu virus.

Since asthmatics tend to become much sicker when they catch the flu, the flu vaccine is recommended yearly for those affected by asthma. In addition, many children with severe asthma take medication that contains corticosteroid as part of their daily treatment. The corticosteroid can further reduce their immune system and make them even more susceptible to infections. This makes the annual administration of the flu vaccine more essential.

Heart Disease

Many children are born with defective hearts. About 1 in 100 children have heart disease at birth. Most of these children have only minor heart problems, but some of them can be gravely ill from their heart defects. A small portion of these children require surgery to allow them to survive past childhood. Having heart defects make these children more vulnerable to certain infections involving the lungs, especially the flu and RSV infection.

The Flu Vaccine

It is recommended that babies born with heart defects are vaccinated against the flu each year because they are more likely to suffer serious complications from the flu. The flu vaccine is normally recommended for children older than six months of age, and it is no exception for children who have heart problems.

Most children with heart defects eventually outgrow their problem. Once their hearts repair themselves, the risk of serious problems when they get the flu is reduced. If your child was born with heart defects, your child's cardiologist should be able to tell you whether he still needs the flu vaccine each year.

The RSV Antibody

Similar to babies born prematurely, infants who are born with serious heart defects are also susceptible to RSV infections. These babies are also recommended to receive the RSV antibody injections during the winter. As these babies grow older, the RSV injections may no longer be necessary. Since each child has a unique heart problem, you need to consult your doctor to find out whether she still qualifies for the RSV injections.

Children Without Spleens

The spleen is an organ that has multiple functions. Aside from recycling old worn-out red blood cells in the body, the spleen is a crucial component of the overall immune system. The spleen filters the blood and constantly looks for the presence of bacteria in the circulating blood. If a germ is detected, it is immediately quarantined and neutralized.

While almost everyone is born with a working spleen, some children and adults end up losing their spleen for one reason or another. A common reason that children lose their spleen is if they have sickle cell anemia. Children with sickle cell anemia have abnormally shaped blood cells. These abnormally shaped cells do not circulate well through the spleen, so over the course of many years the spleen becomes so congested in these children that it eventually stops working. Another reason why children may lose their spleen is if they were involved in a serious accident that caused their spleen to rupture. Surgeons sometimes have no choice but to remove the spleen from these children because these children would otherwise bleed to death. Very few individuals are born without a spleen.

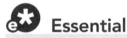 **Essential**

Since children without spleens can get sick so easily, many of them need to take antibiotics on a daily basis to protect their bodies from germ invasion. The routine vaccination for every child is even more crucial in these children without spleens.

Children without a spleen are significantly more prone to getting certain bacterial infections because they lack a crucial component of the immune system. Their bodies are unable to screen out germs from the blood, and bacteria can multiply in their bodies totally unhindered. Currently three vaccines are especially important for these children, including the pneumococcal conjugate vaccine, the Hib conjugate vaccine, and the meningococcal conjugate vaccine.

The Pneumococcal Vaccine

The pneumococcal vaccine is routinely administered to all children at age two months, four months, six months, and again at twelve months of age. For these children without a functional spleen, this vaccine is even more important. Consult Chapter 11 for a more in-depth discussion of the pneumococcal conjugate vaccine.

The Hib Vaccine

The Hib vaccine is already recommended for all healthy children, and children without spleens should receive this vaccine at the same schedule. Recently, there has been a nationwide shortage of the Hib vaccine, and most doctors are skipping some doses of this vaccine to conserve the existing vaccine supply for those who need it the most. If your child has no functional spleen, she must get the complete series of this vaccine. No skipping of doses should be permitted because the risk of life-threatening infection is so high. Please refer to Chapter 10 for more detailed discussion about the Hib conjugate vaccine.

The Meningococcal Vaccine

Meningococcus is a bacterium that can cause devastating infection. The infection caused by this bacterium is particularly aggressive, and it can spread so rapidly that the victim can die on the same day of the first sign of illness. Children without spleens are particularly defenseless against this bacterium, and early vaccination against this infection could be life saving.

The meningococcal conjugate vaccine is not usually recommended for healthy children until early adolescence. However, in children without spleens, this vaccine should be administered at age two years. More recently, there have been research studies that are looking into whether this vaccine could be given at an even earlier age. Please refer to Chapter 16 for more discussion on the meningococcal vaccine. Consult with your child's doctor for the latest recommendation.

Weakened Immune System

A number of conditions can weaken the immune system of children. Some children are born with a weakened immune system, while other children's immune systems may have become weakened by either infections or medications. In any case, these children often require additional vaccines or a modified immunization schedule to compensate for their reduced capacity to protect themselves from germs.

 Alert

In general, children with weak immune systems cannot receive any vaccines containing live germs, including the MMR vaccine, the chickenpox vaccine, and certain types of the flu vaccine. Due to their weakened defenses, the typically innocuous germs in some vaccines can make these children very ill.

Primary Immunodeficiency

Children may have a weak immune system for many reasons. If a child is born with a weak immune system, it is called primary immunodeficiency. This means that nothing has weakened the immune system after birth.

Most primary immunodeficiency occurs in children who have a problem making a particular type of chemical to fight germs. These children derive some protection from germs during the first six months of life because antibody (protective chemicals) from the mother is transferred through the placenta prior to birth to protect the baby. In addition, a breast-feeding mother confers even more protection for her infant because the breast milk contains rich amounts of protective protein that can ward off infections in babies.

Essential

Native American and Alaska Natives are more susceptible to certain infections, including Hib infections, pneumococcal infections, hepatitis A, and hepatitis B. The Hib PRP-OMP conjugate vaccine should be used in these children, and a single-dose of the pneumococcal polysaccharide vaccine should be given after the age of two.

Secondary Immunodeficiency

Secondary immunodeficiency means that the immune system has been weakened after birth. A slew of problems could weaken the immune system in children, including cancers (such as leukemia and lymphoma), chemotherapy for cancers, radiation treatment for cancers, AIDS, medications designed to suppress the immune system (necessary for children who have autoimmune diseases or children who had organ transplantation). Children who have chronic kidney or liver problems also have weakened immune systems because of problems making or retaining protein in the body.

Leukemia and lymphoma are some of the most common childhood cancers. These conditions can lower the immune system because these cancer cells either originate from inside the bones or infiltrate the bones when cancer spreads. In addition to supporting and protecting your body, your bones also serve as the headquarters for your body's defense system. Think of the bones as your body's Pentagon. When cancer cells multiply inside the bones, they squeeze out the normal defense cells in the bones. As these defense cells die out, the overall immune system takes a devastating blow.

Most chemotherapy and radiation regimens are designed to prevent fast-growing cells from multiplying, because cancer cells spread by rapidly making copies of themselves. Unfortunately, today's chemotherapy treatment does not distinguish between multiplying cancer cells and healthy growing cells. When these medications stop cells from multiplying, all the healthy cells that need to grow rapidly in the body are also affected. These include the hair cells, the cells lining the intestines, blood cells, and the immune system cells. Patients undergoing chemotherapy have an extremely weak or nonexisting immune system. They are completely vulnerable to every infection. These individuals need to live in a super-clean environment, and they cannot tolerate getting any vaccines containing live viruses.

Children with AIDS have a weakened immune system because HIV specifically infects immune cells. When immune cells are infected with HIV, they can no longer carry out their usual role of protecting the body. Vaccines containing live viruses can be detrimental for people with AIDS.

People who take corticosteroids because they have conditions that result from chronic inflammation also have weakened immune system. Many children are taking steroids because of severe asthma or allergy problems. Unfortunately, the steroid not only reduces the inflammation in the body, but it also suppresses the immune system.

Finally, people who have had organ transplantations need to permanently restrain their immune system by taking a powerful immunosuppressant. If their immune system is allowed to function unhindered, their body would recognize the transplanted organ as foreign and their immune system would unleash an attack on the foreign organ. This would lead to organ rejection, and death is almost inevitable unless the process can be stopped or they get a new organ. Being in a constant state of immunodeficiency, these patients typically cannot tolerate having live virus injected into their bodies.

Modification to the Immunization Schedule

As mentioned earlier, most vaccines containing live viruses should be avoided by children with defective immune systems. Even though the germs in these vaccines are significantly weakened and pose no threat to healthy children, these germs are nevertheless alive and they can cause life-threatening infection when the immune system is nonexistent or severely weakened. Vaccines that include live viruses are the MMR combination vaccine, the chickenpox vaccine, and the nasal form of the flu vaccine.

Another reason why the immunization schedule needs to be modified for these children is that, due to their underlying problem with their immune system, certain vaccines may not work at all because their immune system cannot be triggered by using traditional vaccines. Administering vaccines to these children would not do them any good, and it exposes them to unnecessary risks. Since the circumstances surrounding each individual is unique, consult your child's doctor for the best strategy to protect your child from infections.

Finally, many children with a weak immune system may require additional vaccines to protect them due to their deficiency. Children without a working spleen especially need protection against germs that can invade their bloodstreams, because the spleen is an important component of the body's defense against germs. Specifically, the Hib conjugate vaccine, the pneumococcal conjugate vaccine, and the meningococcal conjugate vaccine are very important for children without a working spleen. Please consult the earlier part of this chapter for a comprehensive reference if your child has a unique medical condition that may predispose her to certain infections.

CHAPTER 20

Miscellaneous Vaccines

T his book has focused its discussion on the vaccines given to children and adolescents, but there are many other vaccines that are available or in the process of being developed in this country. Some of these vaccines are only used in a particular region of the country, and others are recommended only in special circumstances where an infectious exposure has occurred. Finally, the HIV vaccine is the holy grail of the AIDS scientists.

Introduction

The vaccines discussed in this chapter are not part of the routine childhood immunization program. The Lyme disease vaccine is no longer available in the United States because the vaccine manufacturer stopped making the vaccine in 2002. The rabies vaccine is only recommended for individuals who work with animals or have high risk of being exposed to wild animals. The tuberculosis vaccine BCG is not used in the United States at all, but it is widely used in most other parts of the world. The smallpox vaccine has not been given in this country since 1972. The anthrax vaccine is currently only available to military personnel. Finally, the HIV vaccine has not been invented yet, despite decades of intense research.

The Lyme Disease Vaccine

There used to be a Lyme disease vaccine available in the United States, but GlaxoSmithKline, the company that made the vaccine, stopped producing it in 2002. It was a business decision, and the company cites poor demand for the vaccine as the reason for the cessation. Since that time, no other vaccine manufacturer has decided to make the Lyme disease vaccine.

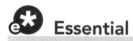 **Essential**

> Transmission of Lyme disease by a tick bite is not common because the tick must stay on the skin continuously for more than twenty-four hours in order to transmit the bacteria in its gut into the blood of the person. Attachment of the tick to the skin for less than twenty-four hours is unlikely to transmit Lyme disease.

Lyme disease is an infection spread by ticks. Not just any tick can spread Lyme disease—only the deer ticks that live mainly in the northeastern, upper Midwest, and mid-Atlantic states. The state of Connecticut has the highest reported rate of Lyme disease, but there have been sporadic cases in northwestern California as well. It appears that the presence of deer is essential for the transmission of the disease.

Lyme disease is a potentially serious infection that can cause chronic arthritis, destruction of the heart muscle, paralysis, and alteration of brain tissue. Fortunately, these serious complications of Lyme disease can be prevented with early treatment of antibiotics. The trick is that the physician must recognize Lyme disease and diagnose the condition in a timely manner in order to institute the treatment without delay.

The Lyme disease vaccine worked fairly well, and it was recommended for people age fifteen to seventy years. Three doses were recommended, and the doses were given over a twelve-month period. The exact duration of the protection offered by the vaccine was not known.

The most common side effects of the Lyme disease vaccine include soreness at the injection site, fever, and mild muscle ache. Serious problems associated with this vaccine have not been reported.

 Fact

In the late 1990s, more than 12,000 people were stricken with Lyme disease. The majority of these patients resided in the northeastern and upper Midwest regions of the United States. Some residents of Canada were diagnosed with Lyme disease as well.

At this point in time, no other American company is planning to make the Lyme disease vaccine. Currently, a version of the Lyme disease vaccine is available for dogs, but humans should not receive this vaccine.

The Rabies Vaccine

The rabies vaccine was one of the earliest vaccines invented. Louis Pasteur, the scientist who discovered bacteria and founded modern microbiology, made the first effective rabies vaccine in 1885. When it was first used on a nine-year-old boy who was mauled by a rabid dog, it most likely saved the life of that boy.

Rabies is a very serious infection that you can get from having direct contact with a rabid animal. Contrary to common belief, you do not have to get bitten by a rabid dog to get rabies. In fact, the most common way to catch rabies in the United States is from handling dead bats or from hunting wild animals, including raccoons, skunks, foxes, and coyotes. Rodents are almost never the vector for rabies. The virus is present in the saliva of the animal, and direct contact with the saliva or brain tissue is necessary to allow transmission.

Once the rabies virus enters the body through large or even microscopic cuts on the skin, it travels slowly through the nerves all the way to the brain. Once the virus reaches the brain, it is always fatal. So far, no treatment has been proven to be consistently effective in reversing the effect of rabies infection once the virus has invaded the brain.

Essential

In the United States, rabies is almost never transmitted from a pet. Almost all cases of rabies in the United States are contracted from contacts with wild animals, especially bats. Domestic animals tend not to harbor this virus in this country.

Rabies is a serious threat in many Asian and African countries. Dogs remain the primary animal harboring the virus in those parts of the world. Each year, more than 50,000 people die from rabies around the world. After being exposed to the virus, a person becomes alternately agitated and depressed and has difficulty drinking fluid (the well-known "foaming at the mouth" sign). Within a weeks time, the person becomes paranoid and hallucinates. Coma is the last stage, and the victim usually dies shortly after.

The rabies vaccine contains weakened but live rabies virus. More than 1.5 million doses of the vaccine have been administered without the report of any serious side effect. Three doses of the vaccine are recommended for people who work closely with animals and are at high risk for getting bitten by animals. If a person has been bitten by a suspected rabid animal, a total of five doses of the rabies vaccine is recommended. So if a high-risk person has already received three doses of the vaccine before getting bitten, only two more doses are needed.

The Tuberculosis Vaccine

The tuberculosis vaccine is called BCG, which stands for Bacillus Calmette-Guérin. This vaccine is not used in the United States, but it is widely used in most other parts of the world. The reason this vaccine is not recommended for Americans is because tuberculosis is not common for people who are born in this country. Most cases of tuberculosis in this country occur among immigrants who may have received the BCG vaccine in their native country.

Question

Why would these immigrants contract tuberculosis even after receiving the vaccine?
The BCG vaccine is not very effective in preventing lung infection caused by tuberculosis. However, it works very well in preventing brain infection caused by tuberculosis. Since brain infection is the most serious form of tuberculosis, this vaccine is still being used in most parts of the world.

The BCG vaccine was first introduced in 1921. However, an early vaccine accident greatly tainted the public image of this vaccine. In 1930, a batch of the BCG vaccine was contaminated with a virulent strain of the tuberculosis bacteria in Germany. Seventy-two babies died from tuberculosis as the result of this vaccine accident. It took more than a decade before this vaccine was gradually accepted by parents again.

Currently, the United States, Great Britain, and Netherlands are the only countries in the world that are not routinely vaccinating against tuberculosis. Great Britain used to have the BCG vaccine as part of its immunization program until 2006, when it decided that the risk of tuberculosis exposure in that country is low enough not to warrant vaccination.

The BCG vaccine contains a live but weakened strain of the tuberculosis bacteria. It is given as an injection. A relatively large scar may form in some people after the vaccination, and occasionally an abscess (a localized infection) may develop at the site of the injection.

Essential

Another reason why the BCG vaccine is not routinely recommended in the United States is that the vaccine can interfere with a screening tool used to test for tuberculosis exposure (the PPD, or purified protein derivative, skin test). The PPD test may turn falsely positive after a recent BCG vaccination.

The Smallpox Vaccine

The smallpox vaccine is the grandfather of all vaccines. Precursors of this vaccine had been used in ancient China for many thousands of years. Even its modern version dates back to the eighteenth century. For a detailed discussion of the history of the smallpox vaccine, please refer to Chapter 1.

There is a resurging interest in this vaccine due to the recent scare of bioterrorism. It is somewhat ironic that recent events have resurrected this ancient vaccine, and now it is relevant in the modern world again. At this time, the smallpox vaccine is only recommended for people in the armed forces in the event of a bioterrorist attack. However, the government currently has enough stockpile of the smallpox vaccine to protect every citizen in this country.

A New Threat

Smallpox has been successfully eradicated after an aggressive global immunization campaign against it. The last death from smallpox occurred in 1978 after a medical photographer was exposed to the virus in a laboratory accident. The director of the laboratory subsequently committed suicide out of guilt. After this accident, the remaining stocks of smallpox virus were destroyed in all laboratories except for two known locations—the high-security laboratory at the Centers for Disease Control and Prevention in the United States and a military laboratory in Russia. Some scientists and government officials worry that the smallpox virus may be hidden in other secret laboratories around the world and could be used as a biological weapon by terrorists. This new concern was the reason why many military personnel and government officials have received the smallpox vaccine in the past few years.

Some people suggest that the remaining frozen sample of smallpox virus should be destroyed at the CDC and Russian laboratories out of fear that the specimen may fall into the wrong hands and be used against civilians in a terrorist attack. The rationale behind keeping this dangerous virus in these laboratories is that scientists may need to learn more about smallpox infection in case such an attack does occur.

Smallpox Infection

There are two forms of the smallpox infection. It could be isolated to the skin or it could spread through the entire body. When the infection affects the whole body, the mortality rate is as high as 30 to 35 percent. Young children have an even higher chance of dying from the infection than adults. Even among the survivors of smallpox, permanent scarring of the skin occurs in 65 to 85 percent of the victims. Blindness and bone infection could complicate a serious smallpox infection.

Smallpox is highly contagious. It is spread from one person to the other through the air, through direct contact, or by contaminated clothing. The infection starts similar to the flu, causing high fevers, headache, and body aches. About two weeks later, the telltale pox lesions appear on the skin. These pus-filled boils then heal gradually in the majority of people, but the disease can progress to the whole body in those who are less fortunate. When the infection becomes wide spread, bleeding from internal organs occurs, and the victim can succumb to the infection rather quickly.

Blindness from scarring on the surface of the eye is a common long-term complication of the infection. In the eighteenth century, a third of all blindness was attributed to smallpox infection. There is no treatment for smallpox, even though vaccination soon after exposure has been shown to lessen the severity of the disease.

The Vaccine

The smallpox vaccine differs from most other vaccines in that it is not given in an injection. Instead, a non-hollow needle is dipped into a liquid solution containing a weakened type of the vaccinia virus, and the needle is then used to puncture the skin several times. A small amount of bleeding can occur with this technique and is considered a normal side effect. The site of vaccination can become sore and quite inflamed afterward. The degree of swelling and redness is generally more dramatic than what you may be used to with a typical vaccination. If the vaccination is successful, a blister forms about a week later at the vaccination site. The blister eventually ruptures and a small scar forms. The sequence of events following vaccination can be scary for those who are not familiar with the process.

Alert

The smallpox vaccine contains live virus, and it is possible to spread the vaccine virus from those vaccinated to those who are vulnerable to it. If you or your child has a weakened immune system, you may not be eligible to get the smallpox vaccine because it can make you quite ill.

The live virus in the smallpox vaccine, called the vaccinia virus, is not the typical smallpox virus. It is not exactly the cowpox virus, either. To this day, it is still unclear how this vaccine strain of the virus originated. Most experts hypothesize that the vaccinia virus is a weakened form of the cowpox virus. Because the vaccinia virus is not the smallpox virus, the vaccine itself cannot give the recipient smallpox.

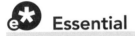 **Essential**

The smallpox vaccine does not offer long-term immunity. Scientists believe that it can offer excellent protection for three to five years, and the immunity wanes after that. A booster vaccine is necessary to remind the immune system and prolong the protection.

Side Effects

The smallpox vaccine is not as safe as most other vaccines recommended for routine childhood immunization. In some people (such as people with pre-existing skin conditions), a severe and life-threatening reaction can occur after vaccination. Children younger than a year old and pregnant women should not receive the smallpox vaccine. The risk of dying from a serious smallpox vaccine reaction is estimated to be one in a million.

The fact that there is a small risk of death and life-threatening complications is the reason why universal vaccination of the entire population is not currently recommended, even in the face of a potential bioterrorism attack. It's all about weighing the risk of the terrorism threat and the risk of the vaccine itself. At this point, the chance of an attack appears to be small.

The Anthrax Vaccine

Shortly after terrorists attacked the United States on September 11, 2001, several letters containing weapon-grade anthrax spores were sent to two U.S. senators and other news agencies. Five people died from anthrax infection, and seventeen others were sickened by the contaminated letters. Even though the casualties were small, it sent a wave of panic and fear throughout the country.

The anthrax bacterium makes an ideal biological weapon. The bacterium is one of the few that can form spores. The biological advantage of having spores is that these spores can remain dormant in a hostile environment for a very long time. Unlike most other bacteria, anthrax spores can remain viable on almost any surface for many decades. Once an unlucky person touches, inhales, or swallows the spores, the spores germinate and the anthrax bacteria spread throughout the body. Even a very small amount of spores can cause a fatal infection. These properties of anthrax spores make it a very effective biological weapon.

Fact

The only shortcoming of anthrax as a biological weapon is that anthrax cannot spread from person to person very easily. Only when a person succumbs to anthrax can his corpse can become a vessel for further transmission. Direct transmission can occur through contaminated clothing, but anthrax outbreak is rare.

Anthrax infection manifests in three forms. If a person contracts the infection by touching the spores, the skin becomes infected and the skin turns black. The infection can subsequently spread to the bloodstream. One out of five people with the anthrax skin infection is expected to die, but antibiotic treatment is most effective for this type of anthrax.

If the spore is inhaled, a person experiences mild fever, shortness of breath, and fast breathing at first. A few days later, almost 100 percent of infected persons die. The inhaled form of anthrax is the most serious and almost always fatal. When anthrax is made into a biological weapon, it is designed to be inhaled by victims, causing the greatest casualties in very short period of time. Even though antibiotic is available for the inhaled form of anthrax, most people die despite treatment.

Finally, if a person swallows the spores in contaminated food, intestinal bleeding, diarrhea, and vomiting of blood result. Half of the people with the intestinal form of anthrax are expected to die. Treatment for intestinal anthrax is available, but the therapy usually is ineffective.

Currently, anthrax is extremely rare in the United States (about a dozen cases are reported annually) due to a mass immunization program for farm animals. Nevertheless, anthrax spores are found in the soil all over the world, including the United States. The most common way of catching anthrax in this country is through direct contact with animal products (such as leather and wool), that are imported from other parts of the world where anthrax remains common.

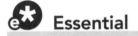 **Essential**

There are more than eighty strains of the anthrax bacteria. Some strains are more aggressive than others, and the most aggressive strains are selected in the laboratory to be made into biological weapons.

The anthrax vaccine was one of the earliest vaccines invented. Back in 1881, French scientist Louis Pasteur (the founding father of modern microbiology) came up with the first working vaccine against anthrax. Since that time, the anthrax vaccine is mainly used in livestock in this country. In 1954, the first anthrax vaccine suitable for humans became available. The only time anthrax vaccine is administered to humans is in the armed forces. American and British soldiers routinely receive a version of the anthrax vaccine to protect them from potential attack in biological warfare.

The HIV Vaccine

Unlike all the other vaccines discussed in this book, the HIV vaccine is unique because no safe and efficacious vaccine has been developed yet. While there are several experimental versions of the HIV vaccine under investigation, none of them have been proven to be effective so far. In previous clinical trials, the investigational HIV vaccines failed to protect recipients from HIV infection.

Acquired immune deficiency syndrome (AIDS) is the infection caused by the human immunodeficiency virus (HIV). The virus directly attacks particular types of immune cells in the body. While HIV does not usually kill its victim directly, the virus decimates the body's defense against other germs, and other infections (such as parasites, tuberculosis, and fungi) take the opportunity to invade defenseless victims and claim the lives of AIDS patients.

The difference between HIV infection and AIDS is that people who are infected with HIV are not diagnosed with AIDS until their immune system has been weakened severely to the point that they become susceptible to many infections. The speed of which the immune system deteriorates depends on a variety of factors—age of the patient, route of transmission, nutritional status, and additional unknown factors. It may take 10 years or more before a person with HIV comes down with AIDS.

Fact

In 2008, the French scientist Luc Montagnier won the Nobel Prize in Medicine for discovering the human immunodeficiency virus and ascertaining its role in causing AIDS. The American researcher Robert Gallo initially claimed that he independently discovered the virus, but it was later found that the virus in Gallo's laboratory was the same one from the French lab.

You may associate HIV infection with certain groups of people—homosexual men and intravenous drug users—but the AIDS global epidemic reveals a different picture. The HIV infection rate in the United States and most developed countries is on the decline, and the vast majority of new infections now occur in Africa. No one is immune to the infection. Heterosexual transmission is most common. AIDS wipes out entire families and villages, frequently leaving helpless orphans behind who are also HIV positive.

HIV infection can be transmitted through unprotected sexual intercourse, breast-feeding, and from the infected mother to her baby during birth. Intravenous drug use is another common way for the virus to spread. Some patients who receive frequent blood transfusions have been infected through contaminated blood in blood banks, but that rarely occurs now since blood donors are carefully screened for the HIV infection.

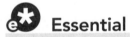 **Essential**

Many people falsely believe that AIDS can be successfully treated with a combination of antiviral medications. While it is feasible to halt the progression of the infection, it is impossible to eradicate the virus completely from the body.

Since the HIV infection is incurable, the best strategy to combat this global epidemic is through preventive vaccination. Prevention via safe sex practices has failed miserably to curb new infections around the world, especially in developing countries. Since the 1980s, about 25 million people have died from AIDS, and the epidemic continues to claim the lives of millions of people each year.

The HIV vaccine was at one point the shining light in the battle with HIV. However, the effort to produce an effective and safe vaccine in the past twenty years has yielded few results, despite an international collaboration in this pursuit. While there are new vaccines that are in the planning stages, it is unlikely that there will be a working vaccine in the near future.

The difficulty with making a working HIV vaccine lies in the fact that the HIV changes constantly. In addition, there are so many subtypes of the virus that a single vaccine cannot possibly protect against so many different variants of the virus. The greatest obstacle yet is to find out how the human body defends itself from the HIV infection. So far, scientists cannot find a reliable mechanism for the immune system to ward off the HIV infection. All previous attempts at coming up with a vaccine have failed miserably.

✅ Fact

In the summer of 2009, a scientific team from the Scripps Research Institute in California announced that they discovered neutralizing antibodies against the virus causing AIDS. This could potentially be the first crucial step in paving the way to developing a vaccine that prevents the HIV infection.

It is possible that scientists may not be able to develop an HIV vaccine for a long time to come. In the mean time, the best strategy against the infection rests on prevention. Condom use is only effective in protecting HIV infection 85 percent of the time, so abstinence is the only way to avoid the infection.

CHAPTER 21

How Vaccines Are Given

This chapter discusses the actual procedure of administering the vaccines. While the details may sound dry and technical, they are nevertheless important to understand. Many parents are unsure of the proper technique of vaccine administration, and they feel uneasy watching the nurses give shots to their children. After you finish reading this chapter, you will have a clear understanding of how vaccines are administered and know whether the nurse is giving the shots correctly.

Storage of Vaccines

First of all, before a vaccine can be administered to your child, the vaccine must be delivered from the vaccine manufacturer to your child's doctor's office and stored properly. A lot of attention is paid to how vaccines are transported and stored. Just like food items and other biological products (donated blood and organs), improper transport and storage can cause a vaccine to become inactive or contaminated. Both conditions pose a serious health threat to your children. Getting a contaminated vaccine can cause infection in the blood stream, which may require your child to be hospitalized.

The federal government has devised exact protocols to ensure proper handling of vaccines during transport and storage so that the vaccines are not damaged or contaminated. Vaccines that do not contain live viruses cannot be frozen during transport and subsequent storage. These vaccines must be refrigerated, however. Vaccines that contain live viruses, including the MMR vaccine, the chickenpox vaccine, and the nasal spray form of the flu vaccine that contains weakened flu virus, must be frozen until they are ready to be administered. Federal inspectors routinely visit doctor's offices to ensure that vaccines are stored properly. This system is set up similarly to the health department inspecting restaurant for food safety.

Essential

The one exception to this rule is the rotavirus vaccine, which does contain live virus. The rotavirus vaccine comes in premixed, single-dose containers, and this vaccine must be refrigerated instead of frozen during transport and storage, unlike all other vaccines that contain live viruses.

Diluent

An additional caveat for many live virus vaccines is that these vaccines are often transported and stored in a freeze-dried state to preserve their effectiveness. This means that these vaccines look like dried powder in their freeze-dried state. Before these vaccines can be administered, they must be mixed with a specially designed liquid, called the *diluent*, to thaw and suspend the powder and activate these vaccines.

While the freeze-dried vaccines must remain frozen during storage, the liquid can be stored at room temperature or in the refrigerator. The diluent must not be frozen or else it would be impossible to mix a frozen block of ice with the dried powder when it is time to activate the vaccine and give the shots.

Each diluent is specifically designed for a particular vaccine. These diluents are not interchangeable, even though they may look similar. If you are concerned about the use of the appropriate diluent for the vaccine, ask your nurse to double-check the diluent while preparing the vaccine for administration.

 Fact

> One exception to the use of the diluent is the Hib conjugate vaccine. Even though the Hib vaccine does not contain live germs, it is also transported and stored in a powder state and must be mixed with a diluent prior to administration.

Light

Many of the vaccines must be protected from prolonged exposure to light during transport and storage. These vaccines can become ineffective when light interacts with the ingredients in the vaccines. The vaccines that must be shielded include the meningococcal vaccine, the MMR vaccine, the chickenpox vaccine, the rotavirus vaccine, and the HPV vaccine. An astute reader may notice that most of the vaccines (but not all) that must be stored in a dark place are live-virus vaccines.

If you are unsure whether your doctor's office is storing vaccines properly, ask the doctor or the nurse to show you where the vaccines are kept in the office. The refrigerator and freezer unit that is used to store medications and vaccines should not contain any food to avoid cross-contamination. A dedicated refrigeration machine should be available for vaccine storage. The temperature of the vaccine refrigerator and freezer should be constantly monitored by a temperature probe that is readily visible at all times. Ideally, an alarm should alert the office staff if the temperature of the refrigeration unit drifts outside of the acceptable range. All office staff working directly or indirectly with vaccines need to be familiar with the proper protocol for vaccine storage.

Vaccine Dose

For many vaccines, single-dose vials are available to allow ease of administration, cut down on dosing errors, and prevent accidental contamination of the vaccine vial. However, these vaccines are obviously more costly to make due to the additional packaging for each dose of the vaccine. Ask your doctor about how the vaccines that your child is getting are supplied.

The amount of liquid given in each injection is the same for most vaccines. Typically, 0.5 ml (milliliter) of the liquid form of the vaccine is drawn up in the syringe and injected. The exceptions include the hepatitis A and hepatitis B vaccine for adults (people older than eighteen years), where 1 ml of the vaccine is injected. Another notable exception is the killed flu vaccine. For children less than three years of age, only 0.25 ml of the vaccine is given. Children older than three receive the same amount of the vaccine (0.5 ml) as adults. Finally, the rotavirus vaccine is an oral vaccine. It comes in single-dose 2 ml vials, and the vaccine is squirted into the child's mouth in its entirety.

Alert

Prior to administering the vaccine, the nurse or medical assistant needs to double-check the expiration date to ensure that the vaccine has not expired. In addition, the lot number of each vaccine, the dose, and the location of administration for each vaccine must be clearly documented in your child's medical record with each vaccination.

Each vaccine must be prepared in the syringe or its own container just before it is given. Drawing up multiple vaccines in advance before they are ready to be given is a bad idea. Once the vaccine is drawn into syringes, they all look the same. It can be impossible to distinguish which syringe contains which vaccine. If multiple vaccines are drawn immediately prior to administration, they need to be clearly labeled so if something happens during the injection process it is known which vaccine was not administered. Giving shots to squirming children is a tough job, and a lot can happen between the time when the vaccine is drawn into the syringe and when the needle hits the skin. An experienced nurse should always be prepared for the unexpected.

If the whole process of transporting, storing, preparing, and charting the vaccination sounds complicated, it is. This is why before each vaccine is given the person administering the vaccine is required by law to double-check with another health-care provider (either another nurse or the doctor) to make sure that no mistakes have been made during the preparation process. Ask your doctor or nurse about the specific protocol that is being practiced at your doctor's office.

Finally, if you want to get the nitty-gritty details of the exact vaccine storage and administration protocol specified by the federal government, you can refer to this site: *www2a.cdc.gov /vaccines/ed/shtoolkit.*

Injection Technique

There have been many studies that looked into the best techniques in giving injection to children to reduce pain. Most vaccines are injected directly into the muscle, while other vaccines must be injected in the fatty tissue under the skin. Those vaccines that are designed for muscular injection include the DTaP vaccine, the Hib conjugate vaccine, the pneumococcal conjugate vaccine, the meningococcal conjugate vaccine, the hepatitis B vaccine, the hepatitis A vaccine, and the HPV vaccine. Vaccines that must be given under the skin include the MMR vaccine, the pneumococcal polysaccharide vaccine, the meningococcal polysaccharide vaccine, and the chickenpox vaccine.

Where the meningococcal vaccine is administered depends on whether the vaccine is the conjugate type or the polysaccharide type. The conjugate vaccine is always given directly into the muscle, whereas the polysaccharide vaccine is given underneath the skin fold. Some vaccines can be given either into the muscle or under the skin. These vaccines include the pneumococcal polysaccharide vaccine and the killed polio vaccine. The nurse giving vaccines should be very familiar with the appropriate techniques for each individual vaccine.

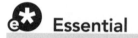 **Essential**

The reason why some vaccines must be given directly into the muscle while others are given under the skin is because certain vaccines work better when they are injected into a particular layer of the tissue. If the vaccine is accidentally the wrong layer, it would not necessarily be harmful, but it may not work as well.

Location of Injection

You must wonder why some people get vaccinated in their buttocks while others receive the injection in their upper arms. If you had a baby recently, you would know that vaccines are usually injected into your baby's thighs. So how do doctors and nurses determine where to give the shots?

It turns out that there are options as to where vaccines can be safely injected into the body. As long as the needle stays away from major arteries and nerves, any site can be used for injection. In addition to avoiding blood vessels and nerves, the location must offer enough tissue so that the needle does not penetrate deep enough to hit bones.

It is generally accepted that the best place to give shots to babies less than a year old is the front of the thigh. There should be plenty of tissue so the needle cannot injure a nerve or blood vessel, and there is no major nerve that traverses through that part of the body.

For older children, the side of the upper arm is typically used for injection because once children are walking, injections in the thigh may cause more pain and interfere with normal ambulation. However, there are times when giving shots on the arm may be difficult or nearly impossible due to a fighting child resisting shots. In these circumstances, injection into the thigh or the buttocks may be necessary.

Speed

Since the number one reason why children fear going to the doctor is shots, it behooves doctors and parents to find out a way to give shots so that they are less painful. In 2007, a study sponsored by American and Canadian doctors looked into whether the speed of the injection mattered with pain perception in children. A standardized pain scale for children was used to determine the degree of pain sensation felt by these children.

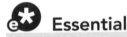 **Essential**

In addition to giving the shots quickly, pinching the skin around the injection site has also been proven to help reduce pain associated with vaccination. If the nurse squeezes the skin of your child, it doesn't mean that she is hurting him. In fact, she is relieving the painful sensation of the injection.

Using the traditional, slower injection approach, the study found that a nurse took an average of eight seconds for each injection. Using the more rapid, needle-in-and-out technique, the nurse took less than one second for each injection. At the end of the study, the scientists found that children experienced significantly more pain with the long, drawn-out injection technique versus the rapid stab technique.

Most experienced nurses already know this, and they always accomplish the vaccination efficiently and quickly. So the next time a nurse quickly gives all the injections to your child, she or he is actually doing your child a favor by stabbing the skin quickly instead of digging in with the needle and taking it out slowly.

Gloves

Many parents are concerned that the person giving the injections does not wear gloves. The act of giving an injection is not a sterile medical procedure, which means the use of gloves is not required. However, it must be done with clean hands, and the location where the skin is punctured by the needle must be cleaned with rubbing alcohol prior to the injection.

☑ Fact

While wearing gloves is not mandatory for the person administering the shots, many people still decide to wear gloves to protect themselves from potential exposure to the small amount of bleeding that may occur with normal vaccination.

Syringe Disposal

The syringe used for vaccine administration is a source of danger, for both children and the adults giving the shots. The syringe must be disposed in the appropriate container immediately after the injection is given. If you see a syringe in the room or on the floor, you must notify the office staff immediately to reduce the risk of puncture injury and potential transmission of infection.

Use of Fever Reducer

Since the majority of children do not experience any fever after vaccination, the use of fever reducers such as acetaminophen

(Tylenol) or ibuprofen (Motrin) are not routinely recommended for everyone after shots. If fever reducers are used for all children every time they get their shots, the majority of children would be taking these medications unnecessarily because they would not have fever reaction anyway.

On the other hand, it is always a good idea to have these medications at home if your child has received vaccination recently. You don't want to be in the position of having a child with a fever in the middle of the night and having to drive all over town to find a twenty-four-hour pharmacy, looking for that one precious bottle of acetaminophen.

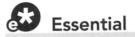 **Essential**

In general, ibuprofen (Motrin or Advil) can cause more side effects than acetaminophen (Tylenol). Stomach ulcers or kidney problems have occurred in children receiving ibuprofen, especially if the child is young or dehydrated. Acetaminophen is a safer alternative for babies less than six months old.

While the fever triggered by vaccination is never harmful, you can certainly give your child fever reducers to make him more comfortable. It is very important to administer the correct dosage of the fever reducer. Calculate the dosage using your child's weight, because children come in all sizes. Using the age alone to calculate the dose can result in underdosing or overdosing. Follow the instruction on the medication packaging carefully, and do not give the medication more often than recommended. Typically acetaminophen (Tylenol) can be given every four hours, and ibuprofen (Motrin) can be given every six hours. It is not a good idea to use both acetaminophen and ibuprofen at the same time. While both medications can be administered safely together, giving both can make it more difficult to keep track of dosing and makes the possibility of overdosing more likely. Call your doctor or a nurse if you are unsure of how much fever reducer to administer.

Developing a relatively high fever is not unusual after vaccination, but a persistent fever should not occur with immunization. A temperature of up to 102°F is not worrisome, but if the fever lasts for more than two days, there might be another reason why your child is having a high temperature. While vaccines are designed to protect your child, they do not protect her from all types of infections. It is entirely possible to get sick from another type of germ (such as croup or a bladder infection) around the time that the vaccines are given. A fever that lasts more than forty-eight hours is the most likely indicator that your child may be sick from something else. Call your doctor if a fever does not go away two days after immunization. For more information on fever and how to manage it, please refer to Chapter 3, on vaccine reaction.

Record Keeping

In the past, immunization records were written by the nurse on a piece of card that the parents keep at home. During each doctor's appointment, the parents were instructed to bring the immunization card so that the doctor could review the record and advise which vaccinations were necessary. While this system worked well most of the time, it was an inefficient system. Occasionally some parents were unable to find the immunization record at home, and sometimes it was difficult to figure out which shots the child had received in the past.

With this system, there was usually a backup record that was also kept at the doctor's office in case the immunization record was misplaced. Having a backup at a doctor's office didn't work all the time because some children changed doctors or relocated to a different area, and it was not always possible to get the information from the previous doctor's office. Every now and then, a doctor retires, and it may be nearly impossible to find the record from the office, even though the government requires that all medical practices keep old medical records for many years without destroying them.

Lost Card

If you cannot find your child's previous immunization record, there is one last place you can look for a copy of the record. Since childhood immunization is recommended by most public schools before attendance, your child's current or previous school may have a copy of the immunization record. While it may not be the most up-to-date record, it may have most of the vaccines your child received prior to age six.

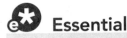 **Essential**

> Even if you are unable to locate your child's immunization record, it is safe to get the vaccines again. Many jobs require an updated copy of your immunization record, especially for health-care workers. No harm has ever been reported for receiving more than the recommended doses of vaccines.

While it is harmless to get all the shots all over again if you have misplaced your child's immunization record, it is nevertheless painful. To avoid putting your child through the discomfort of getting a bunch of additional injections, keep the immunization record in a safe place. To avoid misplacing the record, always keep the card in the same place, preferably with other important documents, such as the birth certificate, the social security card, and passports.

Keep in mind that many childhood vaccines are not necessary anymore for older children, and your child may not need to get all of the vaccines again. Talk to your doctor to find out which vaccines are still necessary for older children.

Electronic Vaccine Record

To circumvent the problem of a misplaced immunization record, most health-care providers are investing in an electronic vaccine tracking system to improve the accuracy of the immunization record and reduce the chance of misplaced records.

Most of these newer systems can still print out a paper copy of the immunization record, and you should keep the paper record in a safe place. While electronic record keeping is more accurate, there is no current accepted national database that contains the vaccine record of all children. If you switch doctors or move away from your current residence, the electronic record at your previous doctor is usually not transferable to the new doctor's office. Unless you have a paper copy of the record to bridge the gap in different systems, missing or duplicate records can become a problem.

Since medical record keeping in general is such an important task, there have been many attempts at creating a national database for individuals to keep their medical records online. Google and Microsoft have independently ventured into this effort, but so far there have been few volunteers who signed on to have their personal information kept online. Obviously, privacy is a major concern and the biggest obstacle to a standardized information system. Until the security details have been worked out and people are convinced that confidentiality will not be breached, such nationwide systems will remain largely underutilized.

CHAPTER 22

Making Decisions

R egardless of what all the statistics and the history of vaccines say, the most important question for you is what is the best thing to do for your child. While this book does not (and cannot) tell you the right thing to do for your unique situation, it does empower you with all the tools and facts you need to make the decision for yourself.

Ethics and Ideals

In the midst of today's vaccine controversy, the frontline of the struggle is often between parents and doctors. Ironically, these are two groups of people who are really striving for the same goal. Everyone wants children to be healthy and grow up to become productive adults. While many parents distrust the medical establishment, there is nothing for the doctors to gain by knowingly poisoning patients with chemicals, not to mention that their own children are among the ones who are immunized. Physicians are not known for being ignorant or lazy. You would think that if there is evidence that suggests there is an unreasonable danger from vaccination, doctors would be among the most vocal opponents of childhood immunization. After all, physicians often lead the way when it comes to reporting dangerous side effects of medications and are always seeking safer alternatives for treatments. Yet the vast majority of physicians (and especially pediatricians) are staunch supporters of childhood immunization. In addition, doctors continue to vaccinate their own children, taking into consideration the risks and benefits of each vaccine.

 Fact

Virtually all pediatricians in the United States vaccinate their own children. If they have any reservation about the safety of vaccines, they would be the first ones to hesitate before having their own children vaccinated.

Another piece of irony is that those who distrust doctors' vaccine recommendations seek out medical advice from the same doctors when it comes to other medical conditions. When their children are experiencing an asthma attack or have injured themselves, parents would not hesitate to go to the same medical establishment that they claim is malicious and ill-informed. After all, the same doctors' organizations and the same group of pharmaceutical companies are endorsing vaccine schedules and treatment for asthma and diabetes. What makes the medical establishment untrustworthy when it comes to vaccination but the pillar of support in treatment of other conditions is difficult to reconcile. It would make more sense that anyone who declines vaccination should forgo all medical treatment for any medical condition, since in their view the medical establishment is either conspiring with the pharmaceutical companies or is too inept to discover blatant flaws in childhood immunization. The same group of healthcare professionals is responsible for recommending immunization for children and treatment for asthma in children. If they are dead wrong in underestimating the risks of vaccination, they could very well make the same mistakes about all medical intervention.

In addition, there is no reason why the government would intentionally poison its citizens. Having a nation of sick and disabled people can place a tremendous burden on a country. You can argue that pharmaceutical companies purposely manufacture unsafe vaccines because of corporate greed or lack of oversight, but these companies are the ones to reap the benefits if the vaccines are proven safe and effective. The threat of lawsuits alone should discourage them from purposely producing harmful products. Protecting innocent children is so intrinsic to human nature that it is hard to imagine any organized institution would openly endorse harmful products for children.

With the best of intentions and knowledge, the medical community supports childhood immunization. It is true that no vaccine is always effective and completely safe, but it is about balancing the risks with the benefits. The vast majority of infections that constantly plague your children are not preventable by vaccines. Only a handful of infections are vaccine-preventable. As a parent, you would do everything possible to protect your child from harm and injury. Just because participation in sports could put your child at risk for serious injuries doesn't mean that you will not allow your child to venture out and engage in athletic endeavors. While vaccine risks are real and present, the risks from disability and death resulting from vaccine-preventable infections are far greater.

Are Vaccines Necessary?

One of the most common questions parents ask is whether any of the vaccines recommended for children today are necessary. After all, humanity survived centuries of warfare with germs and is thriving despite the constant threat of infections. If your ancestors survived their childhood without the help of vaccines, why do your children all of a sudden need to get these foreign chemicals artificially injected into their bodies?

The short answer to the necessity of childhood vaccination is that none of the vaccines are really necessary. If your child never gets exposed to measles, chickenpox, or whooping cough, none of the vaccines would do him any good. Getting children vaccinated would be like preparing to fight an enemy that would never come. The catch is that it is impossible to know whether your child will become the next victim of whooping cough. If you could predict the future, then none of the vaccines would be necessary.

Similarly, car seats are really not necessary. If you and your family never get involved in a car accident, putting your children in car seats or buckling them up in seat belts would be completely unnecessary. In addition, using seat belts and air bags involve their own risks, just like vaccines. Both vaccines and seat belts are preventative measures that are designed to protect in case of an untoward event. If the infection or accident never happens, these measures would be redundant. The only problem is that no one can guarantee that bad things will not happen in the future. There are many things you do to reduce the chance of injury. Seat belts, car seats, and vaccines are among some of the preparation parents can do in anticipating these bad things.

As with the use of seat belts or air bags, vaccines are not risk free. So do you forgo the protection these devices can offer because of the problems associated with them? It all comes down to balancing the relative risk of problems and the potential degree of protection offered by these devices. If you studied the detailed analysis of each vaccine in this book, you can reach your own conclusion about each vaccine.

Since most children are healthy and already have a strong immune system that protects them from germs, many parents question whether vaccination can offer any additional protection against germs. For the same reason that you would want your child to wear a helmet when skateboarding or riding a scooter, you would want as much protection for your child as possible when it comes to serious injuries and infections. Even though your child already has a set of strong bones and skull to protect the brain, you still prefer an extra layer of defense in case of an unanticipated injury. You don't want to leave your child out in the cold when it comes to life-threatening infections, either.

Some parents decide not to vaccinate their children unless there is a community outbreak of the infection. But this practice is flawed. None of the vaccines work fast. Typically it takes between two to six weeks after vaccination before the vaccine can start having a protective effect on a person. In the midst of an infectious disease outbreak, vaccinating children who were previously unprotected would be futile.

Similarly, you would not try to buckle up your seat belt when you realize that an accident is about to occur. There would not be enough time for you to react, and it would be too late by the time you realize you should have worn your seat belt earlier.

The Politics of Immunization

Since childhood immunization is such a significant component of the health-care system, government regulation and control of the program has made vaccines a hot topic in politics. In addition, public schools require parents to show proof of immunization or a statement declining vaccination prior to school admittance. Public health, education, and individual rights become intertwined when it comes to vaccination program and funding.

Political Party

Each political party has a different approach to health care in general. Republicans favor a system where personal responsibility trumps government intervention. Each individual should be responsible for his own health care without big government to put a hand into the matter. This is the reason why government-funded vaccine programs that allow poor families to vaccinate their children get drastically reduced when Republicans are in control of the Congress and White House. Not supporting universal vaccination for children relieves the government of a tremendous financial burden, but if parents do not take the initiative to vaccinate their children and pay for the expenses themselves, the nation could face a greater burden when unvaccinated children become ill with infections.

Democrats believe that the government should play an important role in protecting the health of all children, regardless of wealth or socioeconomic level. Some of the most effective public vaccination programs were instituted by past Democratic presidents. President Franklin D. Roosevelt, President John F. Kennedy, and President Bill Clinton were all strong proponents of childhood immunization, and federal funding for vaccines skyrocketed when they were in the White House. While the upfront cost of these federally funded vaccine programs is staggering, the potential for preventing future health-care costs more than justifies the investment.

Conservatives and Promiscuity

Politicians with a conservative base are against certain vaccines because some vaccines are designed to protect against sexually transmitted diseases. Since sex with more than one partner in a lifetime is not condoned by conservatives, vaccine against sexually transmitted diseases should be completely unnecessary in a perfect world. The HPV vaccine has come under attack by conservatives because opponents say the vaccine undermines the message of abstinence and promotes promiscuity.

Fact

In 2007, Texas became the first state to mandate that all girls entering sixth grade be vaccinated against HPV. The state of Virginia is currently considering such a statewide measure. The legislation is ongoing, and you need to get the most updated information directly from the state legislature.

The problem is that the vast majority of Americans do have more than one sexual partner throughout their entire life. Whether this vaccine was given or not would have very little bearing on people's sexual practice. The vaccine does not protect anyone from all sexually transmitted diseases. So unless we can live in a perfect world, where teenagers never have sex and people never have pre-marital sex, the HPV vaccine will continue to have a role in preventing infections in this imperfect world.

An Issue of Trust

Many people are also wary of the connection between pharmaceutical companies that manufacture vaccines and the government. You may never feel comfortable trusting pharmaceutical companies, yet they are a necessary evil. Without pharmaceutical companies, your child would have no antibiotics to treat a life-threatening infection. If you truly mistrust pharmaceutical companies and doctors, you may have to be wary of the entire health-care system, not just vaccines. The same people who make the vaccines also make antibiotics and other medications, and the same doctors who recommend immunization for your child are also the ones who treat your child when she is sick. How can you trust the same group of people in one circumstance and not in another? If doctors are lazy and ignorant (or just plain malicious), there is no one to turn to except yourself when your child gets sick.

Parental Rights

The only circumstance when parents lose their rights to be their children's surrogate is when the parents knowingly and intentionally put their children in harm's way or abandon the children. Parents are supposed to be the most trusted advocate for their children's best interests. When there is evidence of neglect or abuse, this sacred right is removed by the legal system.

✪ Essential

Virtually all the states in America allow parents to refuse vaccination for personal or religious reasons. Only two states—Mississippi and West Virginia—do not allow parents to decline vaccines. In these states, the only reason a child can skip routine vaccination is due to a documented medical reason.

When parents refuse vaccination for their children, they are not acting out of malice or with any intent to harm. They are being their children's advocate, and they are doing everything possible to protect their children from harm. This important legal right should be respected, and government officials and physicians should understand the intention of parents. The right thing to do is not to deprive these parents of their rights but to make sure that they have the most reliable and up-to-date information when they make their decision for their children's health. Generally speaking, the government and doctors are not doing enough to understand the perspective of these parents and provide them with information. A more punitive approach is usually employed, and this only makes some parents more defensive.

✅ Fact

Some states have laws that mandate vaccination for attendance of public schools. Consult your state legislature for such information. This book does not provide the information because it is impossible to stay current on the constantly shifting legal landscape.

In addition to vaccines, parents also have the right to refuse treatment for their children. As long as withholding treatment does not have a high probability of causing disability or death, most doctors should respect the parental wish. If a parent stands in the way of a life-saving medical intervention, doctors can supercede parental rights and administer the necessary treatment. If time permits, a court order should be obtained by the treating physician before overriding parental wishes.

Ultimately, neither the government nor health-care professionals should tell people what to do with their bodies, even in the name of protecting them. Each individual should retain the right to make decision about his own health. The government can and should protect minors when they are not capable of making decisions for themselves due to their youth. This is already an accepted role of the government. Current laws prohibit the sale and advertisement of cigarettes to minors but not to adults. Adults already possess enough life experience and wisdom to make decisions on their own, even if their action causes them harm. The government and health-care professionals should educate the public so each adult citizen can make the best decision based on the best available information. If a well-informed citizen decides to poison his body with cigarettes, it's perfectly legal.

Herd Immunity

Vaccines do not work 100 percent of the time. Due to this shortcoming, a community can only be protected if the majority of the people are immunized. When a large segment of the community has not received vaccination, even those who are immunized are vulnerable to these infections and community outbreaks. You cannot skip vaccinating your children and just count on your friends and neighbors to vaccinate theirs. They might be counting on you to have your children vaccinated so they don't have to vaccinate theirs.

Eventually, everyone would be hoping that everyone else would vaccinate their children, and no one would be vaccinated in the community. You also know now that vaccination comes with some risks. If no one wants to take on that risk with their own children, then ultimately no one would be vaccinated and the entire community would be vulnerable to infectious outbreaks and everyone suffers. The consequences of having outbreaks spreading through the entire society are ominous, and the world your children will live in would not be so different from your grandparents' more than fifty years ago, when whooping cough and polio claimed thousands of lives and maimed even more.

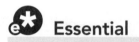 **Essential**

Many vaccine opponents point out that children who are vaccinated can still get sick from the infection vaccines are supposed to prevent. This is completely true. Vaccines do not work 100 percent of the time. It is also fair to say that virtually nothing man made works 100 percent of the time, but it doesn't mean that you'll stop driving your car or using your refrigerator.

In many ways, every child is in this together. You either take on a small risk by vaccinating your children (and hoping that your neighbors do the same), or the entire community suffers, including your children. Your children's future is in your hands. What you do and don't do right now can affect generations of children to come. Keep in mind that the people affected will not just be other people's children but your children and grandchildren and great grandchildren.

It is still not an easy decision, given that vaccines are not risk-free and serious side effects can change your child's life forever. But if every parent decided not to vaccinate, the future will indeed be very dark and grim for humanity. The world will gradually drift back into a time when infectious diseases claim young lives regularly and randomly.

Your Child, Your Choice

When it comes down to it, the buck stops at your feet. You are ultimately responsible for providing your child with the best possible future, and you are ultimately responsible for creating the safest surrounding so your child can thrive to her highest potential. All that doctors and the government should do is support you in this effort. No one should tell you what to do.

If you elect not to vaccinate your child, there is a chance your child can get sick from any of the vaccine-preventable diseases circulating in the community. The most common infections that are still prevalent in the United States are whooping cough, rotavirus, and influenza, and there are sporadic measles outbreaks. You can protect your child without resorting to immunization by minimizing the exposure to infectious diseases. Home schooling would be recommended until age twelve, daycare is out of the question, and any participation in group activities with other children should be avoided. Crowded public places, including the supermarket, the library, and public playgrounds, are breeding grounds for germs, and so these places must be avoided whenever possible.

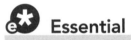 **Essential**

If you choose not to vaccinate your children, you must breast-feed for at least the first twelve months to transfer additional chemicals from the breast milk that can be critical in protecting your baby from germs. If you are unable to breast-feed for the first year, you should seriously reconsider your decision not to vaccinate.

If you still cannot make up your mind about immunization after reading this book, what else can you do to prepare yourself for this daunting but important decision? You need to keep an open mind and arm yourself with knowledge—not information from anywhere, but reliable information. Be wary of what you read on the Internet and see on the television. What do they know about vaccine safety? How do you verify the source of the information?

The best and most reliable information is from a trained health professional you can trust. Don't settle for any doctor; shop around and find one who is willing to listen to you and answer your questions. If a doctor starts telling you that you must do this or that without giving you the information to let you make up your own mind, you need to find another doctor. A good doctor is one who will take the time and understand your perspective. A good doctor understands that the most important ally in providing the best care for your child is you. A good doctor works with you. Your job is to find such a trustworthy health-care ally and make the decision together for your child.

Current Recommended Immunization Schedule

At the time this book was written, the childhood immunization schedule was as follows. Consult your pediatrician for the most up-to-date immunization schedule for your child.

- **Hepatitis B:** first dose at birth, second dose within the first two months after birth, and the third dose at four to six months of age.

- **Rotavirus:** first dose at two months, second dose at four months, and third dose at six months. This vaccine cannot be given after eight months of age.

- **DTaP:** first dose at two months, second dose at four months, third dose at six months, fourth dose between twelve and eighteen months, and the last dose at four years.

- **Hib:** first dose at two months, second dose at four months, third dose at six months, and the fourth dose is recommended between twelve and eighteen months if there is no vaccine shortage.

- **Pneumococcal conjugate:** first dose at two months, second dose at four months, third dose at six months, and the fourth dose is recommended between twelve and eighteen months.

- **Polio:** first dose at two months, second dose at four months, the third dose between six and eighteen months, and the fourth dose at four years.

- **Flu (injectable):** starting from six months of age, annually from September to June. If the first dose is given before the age of nine, a booster shot is recommended for the first flu season.

- **MMR:** first dose at one year (must be administered after the first birthday), and the second dose at four years.

- **Chickenpox:** first dose at one year (must be administered after the first birthday), and the second dose at four years.

- **Hepatitis A:** first dose at one year, and the second dose at least six months after the first dose.

- **Meningococcal:** during adolescence, but may be given to children as young as two years

- **HPV:** three doses given six months apart starting from age nine for girls.

Finding More Information on Immunization

Even though this book does not recommend parents get vaccine information from the Internet, you may still find these websites useful. The best source of information on vaccines is from a doctor that you know well and trust.

Immunization information from the American Academy of Pediatrics offers up-to-date information on some of the newest vaccines on the immunization schedule.
www.cispimmunize.org

The Pennsylvania Chapter of the American Academy of Pediatrics provides additional information on childhood immunization. It has a detailed section that answers the most common questions regarding vaccine safety.
www.paiep.org

Vaccinate Your Baby is an organization that raises awareness of various vaccine controversies and provides an informational guide directed toward parents who are faced with the decision of whether to vaccinate their children.
www.vaccinateyourbaby.org

Immunization information from the World Health Organization gives a global perspective on infection control and offers the latest data in vaccine research. It also has a comprehensive section that provides advice on vaccination for travelers.
www.who.int/immunization/topics/en

The Centers for Disease Control and Prevention website handles vaccine information that is most relevant to families living in the United States.
www.cdc.gov/vaccinesafety

The Children's Hospital of Philadelphia has a website that is frequently updated and gives a parental perspective on childhood immunization.
www.chop.edu/consumer/your_child/index.jsp

Immunization Action Coalition is a website that is designed primarily for doctors, but if you have a medical background or would like to get vaccine information from a scientific perspective, you may find this site useful.
www.immunize.org

Johns Hopkins School of Public Health maintains this website, which has the most comprehensive information on vaccine components and preservatives.
www.vaccinesafety.edu

The National Network for Immunization Information provides facts about immunization. It is a good place to start if you are interested in the more technical aspect of vaccines.
www.immunizationinfo.org

You can download your copy of the Vaccine Information Statements from the CDC at the following URL. The VIS papers are the handouts that are provided by your doctor at each office visit when your child gets vaccinated.

www.cdc.gov/vaccines/pubs/vis/default.htm

You may use Google or another search engine to find more information on the web, but be wary of any website that advertises books or herbal supplements. These websites are designed primarily to sell you products and may not have the most reliable information.

In addition to the Internet, there are many other books that can provide you with a different perspective on vaccines. Once again, the best resource for vaccine information is still your trusted doctor. The following is a list of books that may be helpful.

Vaccine: The Controversial Story of Medicine's Greatest Lifesaver, Arthur Allen. 2008, W. W. Norton.

Vaccinations: A Thoughtful Parent's Guide: How to Make Safe, Sensible Decisions about the Risks, Benefits, and Alternatives, Aviva Jill Romm. 2001, Healing Arts Press.

Do Vaccines Cause That?!, Martin Myers and Diego Pineda. 2008, Immunizations for Public Health.

Autism's False Prophets: Bad Science, Risky Medicine, and the Search for a Cure, Paul Offit. 2008, Columbia University Press.

APPENDIX C

Frequently Asked Questions

1. **Since many infections preventable by vaccines are so rare now, why is it still necessary to vaccinate children against these diseases?**

   While measles, polio, and hepatitis have become uncommon in the United States, these infections still pose a threat to American children because of air travel and the world being much more connected than ever before.

   Past outbreaks that started with a particular infection could only spread so far because transportation of the infected people was limited. While virtually all cases of measles and polio in the United States today are imported, an outbreak within the country would occur if the majority of American were not immunized against these infections because we are more connected and not limited by travel. The only reason why these infections remain rare in this country is because of the existing public immunization program.

2. **Are vaccines safe? How do you know that vaccines are harmless?**

   In fact, vaccines are not completely safe. Just like every medical intervention and treatment, there are small risks involved, and vaccination is no exception.

Many routines that you carry out daily have definite risks involved. Driving your child around, feeding your child solid foods, bringing your child to a birthday party—all involve potentially fatal complications. More children die from motor vehicle crashes than any other reason. Choking is a very real and common risk for young children, and cooking food in the kitchen poses significant risk for serious burn injury for your child. A food allergy can be life threatening for some children, and the reaction is completely unpredictable. Latex balloons, common at birthday parties, are the most common cause of choking death for children. Danger is everywhere around your child, so how can you minimize the risks?

There is no question that you still need to feed your child and drive your child around. These activities are unavoidable, but it doesn't mean you give up doing them completely just because they involve certain risks. Obviously, the risk of starvation and death is much greater than from food allergy and choking, so you feed your child despite the risks.

Vaccination is the same way. There is definite risk involved, but not vaccinating carries risks as well. For all childhood vaccines, the risk of being hurt from the vaccines is far smaller than the risk of being injured from the infections themselves. So you have to pick the lesser of the two evils and accept the calculated risk of vaccination.

Remember, not doing something can actually be more dangerous. Not buckling up your children in seat belts can cause more harm.

3. **Do vaccines work at all? Many people say that the reduction in infectious diseases in the last few decades is the result of improved sanitation and a higher standard of living.**

Better sanitation and improvement in the standard of living do make a significant impact on infection control. However, many of the infections that are now rare did not become uncommon until the late 1980s, when vaccines against these infections became available. Sanitation and the standard of living did not change drastically from the 1980s to the 1990s, and the vaccine is most certainly the reason why these infections are uncommon today.

4. **Do healthy children with a strong immune system really need vaccines to protect them from infections?**

Many parents would rather rely on their children's own immune system to fight off infection naturally than on artificial vaccines. Why inject all these foreign chemicals into the body when the body is already equipped with its own defense system to ward off germs?

It is true that most children can fight off germs on their own, but not every child is so lucky. Many children who suffer permanent injuries from infections have healthy immune system, but they get gravely ill anyway. If the germs are particularly aggressive, even the best natural immune system cannot prevent a frontal attack by some germs.

Relying on your child's own immune system is like relying on your child's own skull in case of an accident. Why wear a helmet when riding a scooter or bike when your child is already equipped with a very hard skull?

5. **Can all these dead germs being injected into the body at the same time overwhelm your child's immune system?**

There are germs everywhere—on the surface of the skin, in the nose, and inside the intestines. If your child attends daycare, the whole place is literally crawling with germs. Every time your child eats or drinks anything, she is swallowing germs because the foods are not sterilized.

The human body is designed to handle hundreds of thousands of germ attacks constantly, and if a handful of shots can overwhelm the immune system, the human species would have become extinct a long time ago.

6. **Do vaccines weaken the immune system because vaccination deprives the body's opportunity to fight off infections naturally?**

Vaccines are designed to boost the immune system before a real encounter with an infection. The benefit of vaccines is that your child's immune system can be bolstered without risking getting the detrimental effect of natural infections. Instead of weakening the body, vaccination enhances the body's natural defenses.

7. **If a child has a cold, can she still get vaccinated?**

Routine vaccination should be postponed when a child is suffering from a serious illness. Serious illness is defined as a condition that significantly alters the body's normal functions. If your child has a high fever (temperature greater than 102°F), is lethargic or severely dehydrated, or needs to be hospitalized due to the severity of an illness, immunization should be postponed.

However, if your child has a cold or minor viral infection, routine vaccination can proceed safely.

8. If your child accidentally gets an extra dose of a vaccine, is it harmful?

While getting an additional dose of a vaccine beyond the standard recommended schedule does not make it work better, it is not harmful or dangerous. The brief pain and discomfort associated with the injection notwithstanding, the additional vaccine would not disrupt the immune system.

If you want to prevent your child from getting more vaccines than necessary, you should keep track of all of your child's immunization records so duplication of vaccines would not occur.

9. How do I report vaccine side effects?

Anyone can report reactions that occurred after vaccination to the Centers for Disease Control and Prevention and the Food and Drug Administration directly. The Vaccine Adverse Event Reporting System (VAERS) is an extensive computer system designed to collect and track possible side effects caused by vaccines.

If your child experiences any unusual reaction following immunization, you can report the reaction by filing a report online at *http://vaers.hhs.gov*

Any reaction observed following vaccination can be reported to VAERS, no matter how mild. As a result, the majority of reports include minor symptoms such as low-grade fever, pain at the vaccine injection site, and headaches.

Keep in mind that not all reactions reported to VAERS are actually caused by vaccines. If a child falls off his bike a day following routine vaccination and gets a nosebleed, the nosebleed can be reported to VAERS, even though most people would agree that the vaccine probably did not trigger the nosebleed. Remember, any event that occurs following vaccination is reported to VAERS.

Glossary

adjuvant: A chemical frequently added to vaccines to enhance the effectiveness of the vaccine. A common adjuvant in many vaccines is aluminum.

AIDS: Short for acquired immune deficiency syndrome, it is the end-stage infection caused by the human immunodeficiency virus (HIV). By the time a person is diagnosed with AIDS, he has little or no immunity against many germs.

anaphylaxis: A serious allergic reaction involving the whole body. Unless medical intervention is quickly instituted, the reaction can be fatal.

antibiotic: A substance used to treat infections caused by bacteria. Antibiotics do not work at all against infections caused by viruses.

antibody: A chemical made by your immune system that targets a specific type of germ. Most vaccines are designed to trigger the body's immune system to generate a particular type of antibody against a germ.

congenital rubella syndrome: A deformity and disability in the baby that results from a rubella infection in the mother during pregnancy. Blindness, deafness, mental retardation, and heart defects are common features of congenital rubella syndrome.

efficacy: How well something works. When applied to vaccines, it means how well the vaccine works to prevent an infection.

encephalitis: Infection of the brain tissue. People with brain infections are agitated or confused, or they could become comatose.

Guillain Barré Syndrome: A neurological condition that is caused by inflammation of the nerves in the spinal cord. Temporary paralysis of the arms and legs can result from this condition.

herd immunity: The concept that vaccines work better when the majority of the people in a community are immunized. Since vaccines do not always work, the only way the entire community can be protected from infectious outbreaks is from herd immunity.

Hib: Short for *Haemophilus influenzae* type b, which is a type of bacterium that used to be the most common cause of bacterial meningitis in children. This bacterium can also cause a life-threatening throat infection, joint infection, bone infection, and skin infection.

HPV: Short for human papilloma virus, a sexually transmitted disease. This virus is responsible for causing almost all cervical cancer. A vaccine made available in 2006 protects women from this virus.

immunoglobulin: An antibody that can be given to a sick person to help the person fight off an infection. Immunoglobulin is very expensive, and it is only used if the person is gravely ill or if there is no other treatment available.

immunosuppressed: A state where one's immune system is weakened for a variety of reasons. Diseases, infections, or medications can all cause immunosuppression in people.

inflammation: Irritation of a part of the body, usually identified by redness, swelling, pain, and warmth.

meningitis: Infection of the thin covering of the brain. If the infection is caused by bacteria, it is usually much more serious and the fatality rate is much higher. If the infection is caused by viruses, the infection is less devastating. A spinal tap (lumbar puncture) is necessary to confirm the diagnosis.

meningococcus: A bacterium that can cause meningitis and blood infection in children and adolescents.

pandemic: An infection that affects a large number of people over a large area. Usually multiple countries are involved in a pandemic.

pertussis: The scientific term for whooping cough.

pneumococcus: A bacterium that frequently causes pneumonia, blood infection, and ear infection in children. This bacterium also caused a large number of bacterial meningitis before a vaccine against it was available.

pneumonia: Infection of the lung tissue.

Reye's syndrome: A life-threatening reaction that is characterized by inflammation of the liver, swelling of the brain, and ultimately death. The reaction occurs when a child with the flu or chickenpox is given aspirin.

rotavirus: A stomach virus that causes the majority of diarrhea in babies.

RSV: Short for respiratory syncytial virus, which is a type of virus that causes runny nose, cough, and fever in young children. Adults can get sick from RSV, but the illness is usually much milder, and often indistinguishable from the common cold

rubella: The scientific term for German measles. This infection is harmless except when a pregnant woman gets infected. The fetus usually becomes deformed from the infection.

shingles: Chickenpox virus that has awakened from a dormant state in the body, causing a group of painful blisters to appear on a patch of skin. Shingles usually affect only one side of the body.

SIDS: Short for sudden infant death syndrome; it occurs when a baby less than a year old dies from no apparent reason.

strain: Similar but not different enough to merit a new species name; often used to describe types of germs.

thimerosal: A mercury-based preservative that was once commonly used in childhood vaccines. Thimerosal was removed from all childhood vaccines in 2001.

varicella: The medical name for chickenpox.

variolation: An old and out-dated technique that was used to introduce a small amount of smallpox virus into a healthy individual. Variolation protects the person from future smallpox infection, but the process itself also carries significant risks. Some people who were variolated ended up dying from the variolation procedure.

Index